OVER 50 *DIET*

**THIS BOOK INCLUDES:
KETO DIET** *and* **INTERMITTENT FASTING
FOR PEOPLE 50+
AN EASY GUIDE WITH RECIPES FOR
HEALTHY WEIGHT LOSS, BURN FAT** *and* **SLOW AGING**

Amanda K. Loss

@ Copyright 2020 by Amanda K. Loss - All rights reserved.

This Book is provided with the sole purpose of providing relevant information on a specific topic for which every reasonable effort has been made to ensure that it is both accurate and reasonable. Nevertheless, by purchasing this Book you consent to the fact that the author, as well as the publisher, are in no way experts on the topics contained herein, regardless of any claims as such that may be made within. As such, any suggestions or recommendations that are made within are done so purely for entertainment value. It is recommended that you always consult a professional prior to undertaking any of the advice or techniques discussed within.

This is a legally binding declaration that is considered both valid and fair by both the Committee of Publishers Association and the American Bar Association and should be considered as legally binding within the United States.

The reproduction, transmission, and duplication of any of the content found herein, including any specific or extended information will be done as an illegal act regardless of the end form the information ultimately takes. This includes copied versions of the work both physical, digital and audio unless express consent of the Publisher is provided beforehand. Any additional rights reserved.

Furthermore, the information that can be found within the pages described forthwith shall be considered both accurate and truthful when it comes to the recounting of facts. As such, any use, correct or incorrect, of the provided information will render the Publisher free of responsibility as to the actions taken outside of their direct purview. Regardless, there are zero scenarios where the original author or the Publisher can be deemed liable in any fashion for any damages or hardships that may result from any of the information discussed herein.

Additionally, the information in the following pages is intended only for informational purposes and should thus be thought of as universal. As befitting its nature, it is presented without assurance regarding its prolonged validity or interim quality. Trademarks that are mentioned are done without written consent and can in no way be considered an endorsement from the trademark holder.

TABLE OF CONTENTS

Book #1: KETO DIET OVER 50 - *The Ultimate and Complete Guide for Healthy Weight Loss, Slowing Aging and Preventing Diabetes with Ketogenic Lifestyle+ 10-Day Meal Plan with 30 Low-Carb Recipes*..9

Introduction..11

Chapter 1: What Is the Ketogenic Diet?....................................13
    Types of Ketogenic Diets.. 20
    Some Side Effects to Lookout For... 21

Chapter 2: Benefits of the Ketogenic Diet.............................23
    Natural Weight Loss 24
    Hunger Management.. 27
    More Energy and Mental Clarity 30
    Boosted Brain Health with Keto 34

Chapter 3: Side Effects and Do's and Dont's........................37
    Fatigue and Dizziness 38
    Constipation... 39
    Sugar Cravings 39
    Shakiness or General Weakness 40
    Kidney Stones 40
    Racing Heart 41
    Low Carb Flu or Keto-Flu 42
    Intake of Too Many Carbs.. 47
    Intake of Too Much Protein 47
    Low Sodium Levels 48

Chapter 4: Ketogenic Diet for Younger People vs Older People..................51
Bone Health 54
How the Keto Diet and Ketosis Is Important for Aging 58
Using Ketosis to Achieve Longevity.......................... 60

Chapter 5: Ketogenic Diet and Working Out......................61
Resistance Training is Key................................ 64
Sets, Repetition, Tempo..................................67
Reading Tempo Breakdown 68
Tempo Breakdown for Beginners............................. 69
How Sets Are Used for Different Goals 69
Primal Movements 70
Squat Regression to Progression 72
Rowing/Pull-ups Regression to Progression 73
Push-Ups Regression to Progression.........................75
Hinge/Deadlift 76
Planks/Abdominal Work................................... 78
Resistance Training for General Population 80

Chapter 6: How to Make This a Lifestyle........................87
Plan Your Day Ahead 88
It Will Help You Prioritize............................... 88
More Focus on the Task in Hand 89
Work-Life Balance... 89
Summarize Your Normal Day 90
Arrange Your Day...91
Remove All the Fluff.......................................91
Be Grateful... 92
Stop Multitasking 96

Chapter 7: 10-Day Eating Plan + Recipes **103**
   Breakfast 106
   Lunch 113
      Salads.. *113*
      Pasta *121*
      Pizza...*126*
      Tacos & Wraps..*132*
   Dinner 135
      Beef for Dinner *135*

Conclusion..**153**

BOOK #2: INTERMITTENT FASTING *OVER 50* -
The Ultimate and Complete Guide for Healthy Weight Loss, Burn Fat, Slow Aging, Detox Your Body and Support Your Hormones with the Process of Metabolic Autophagy..157

Introduction..159

Chapter 1: What Is Intermittent Fasting?..................161

Chapter 2: Benefits of Intermittent Fasting..................171

Chapter 3: Different types of fasting protocol..................187

Chapter 4: How to Pick the Right Plan Based on Your Lifestyle..203

Chapter 5: How Does Intermittent Fasting Slow Down Aging..215

Chapter 6: How Should Women Fast Over 50?..................225

Chapter 7: Manage the Symptoms of Menopause..............245

Chapter 8: Recipes + 10-Day Plan..................257
    Breakfast..259
        Crustless Broccoli Sun-dried Tomato Quiche..................259
        Chocolate Pancakes..................................262
        Breakfast Scramble..................................264
        Superfood Breakfast Bars..................................266

Lunch 268
- Vegan Tuna Salad 268
- Veggie Wrap with Apples and Spicy Hummus 270
- Mac and Cheese Bites 272
- Chick'n Salad with Cranberries and Pistachios 274

Dinner 276
- Pan-fried Jackfruit over Pasta with Lemon Coconut Cream Sauce 276
- Butternut Squash Tacos with Tempeh Chorizo 279
- Vegan Fish Sticks and Tartar Sauce 281
- Vegan Philly Cheesesteak 284

Desserts and Snacks... 286
- Mango Lime Chia Pudding 286
- Mint Chocolate Truffle Larabar Bites...................................288
- Peanut Butter Caramel Rice Krispies 290
- Easy Chocolate Pudding.. 292

Conclusion..**295**

KETO DIET OVER 50

*The Ultimate and Complete Guide
for Healthy Weight Loss, Slowing Aging
and Preventing Diabetes
with Ketogenic Lifestyle
+ 10-Day Meal Plan with 30 Low-Carb Recipes*

INTRODUCTION

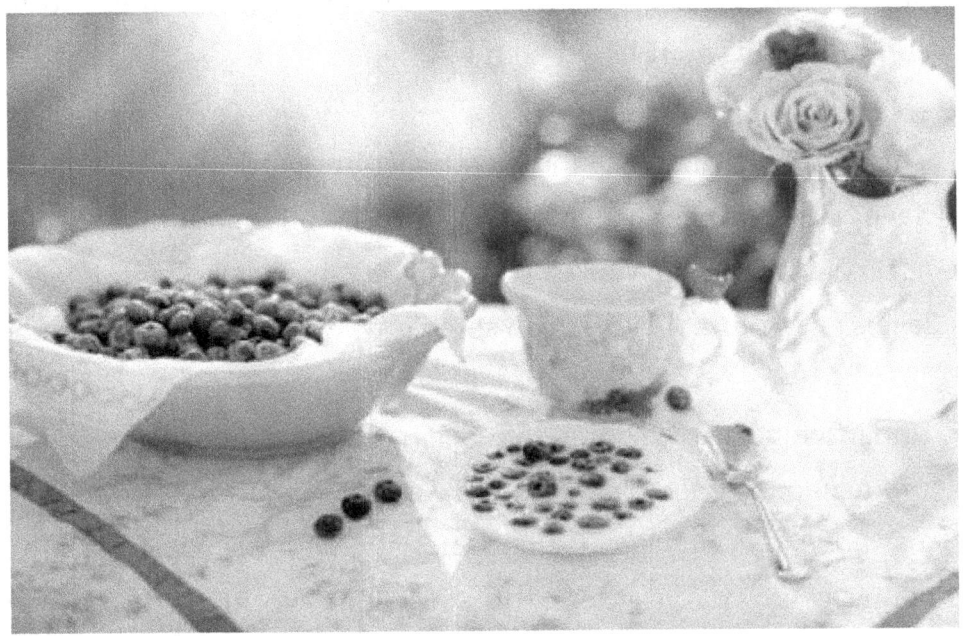

Thank you so much for choosing this book *Keto Diet Over 50*. We will show you how to make your Ketogenic diet journey amazing and hassle-free.

If you are reading this, it is because you are keen on learning more about how you can improve your overall health and wellbeing while dropping some pounds along the way. So, this book has been written with you in mind. It doesn't matter where you are coming from. What truly matters is that you are concerned about improving yourself.

In this book, you will find tips and strategies regarding the use of the ketogenic diet as a means of losing weight, feeling better, and improving your health and wellbeing.

This book isn't about another one of those fad diets that don't have any science backing them. It is all about a sensible approach in which you can improve your metabolism, energy levels and your ability to keep some unwanted extra pounds off.

In particular, we are going to focusing on *how the ketogenic diet can help older folks find a balance between their overall weight loss goals and their wellbeing.* And while it is also useful for the younger crowd out there, the fact that we are going to be focusing on the ketogenic diet for older folks makes this book highly specialized.

So, what are you waiting for?

Come on in and let's get started today on your personal journey to improving your health and wellbeing!

Chapter 1: What Is the Ketogenic Diet?

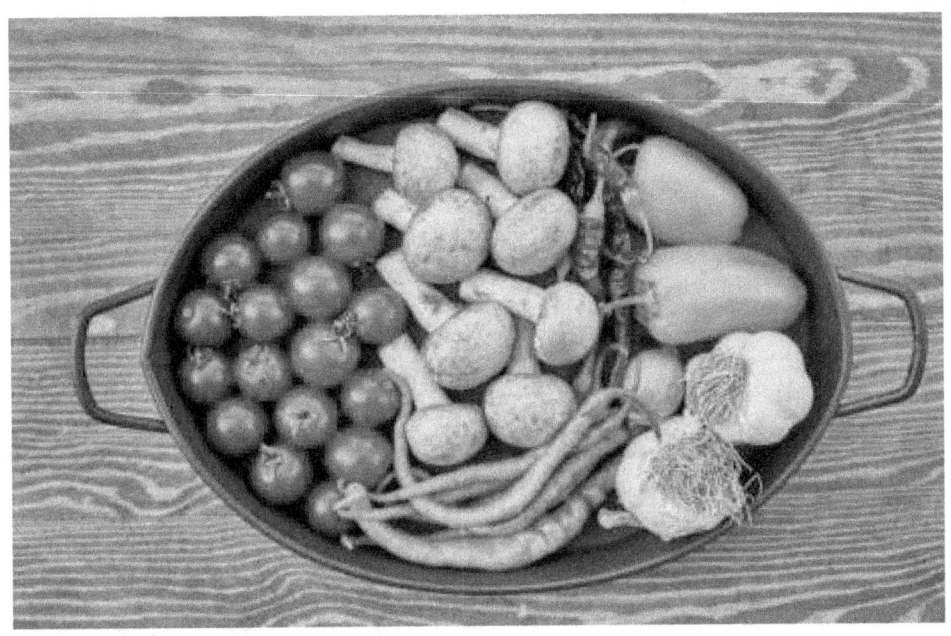

Hundreds of years ago, what we ate did not matter that much because we were healthy as we only ate natural foods available. However, over the decades, the food industry transformed, and food companies started introducing food additives and chemicals to food to increase its taste and shelf life.

This transformation resulted in an increase of diseases previously unheard of in ancient times. In this book, you will learn what this diet is, how it works, its benefits, and how you can adapt it to have a lean body free from excess fat and live a healthy life. Obesity becomes one of the scariest words in the modern world. Being overweight has become an annoying problem. Many people are trying to lose their weight by following many kinds of dieting methods. Since an ideal bodyweight and a healthy body condition are significant concerns nowadays, the diet has become a trend in the new community.

Many people have tried many dieting methods with all of their hard treatments. Even, some people are willing to pay handsomely to reach the ideal bodyweight. You might have heard that a Ketogenic diet is a dieting method that has been effective for the last several years. It is also known as a Low Carb Diet.

Principally, the Ketogenic diet involves a high intake of fat, moderate consumption of protein, and tremendously low eating of carbohydrates. In other words, it can be said that the Ketogenic diet is a dieting method that encourages the liver to produce more ketone bodies. Lucky you, this book provides many recipes that will help you to prepare excellent and healthy food! In this book, you will learn valuable and critical information on how you can use the Ketogenic diet to lose weight and better your health.

The Ketogenic diet is a diet that focuses on reducing your carbohydrate intake and makes you eat more healthy fats. It is also a diet that has been proven not only to help lose pounds but also to control significant medical conditions like epilepsy. In the following chapters, we will explain exactly what the Ketogenic entails, how it is different from other diet plans, the benefits, and some helpful guidelines on what to eat and what to avoid when living a Ketogenic lifestyle. This book will teach you everything you need to know about the Ketogenic diet, how it works, what foods to eat, what foods to avoid, and how you can get started. This book also contains a starting 10-day keto meal plan that can help guide you through your very first phase. Starting a keto diet can be tough if you don't have a good idea for what to eat. That's where this 10-day keto meal plan comes in. We've done all the calculations, cooking, and planning for you. Now you can relax and enjoy all the benefits of a Ketogenic diet stress-free. Thank you again for believing in us and getting started. I hope that you will enjoy it and that it'll help you along your journey to more excellent health.

I am so excited that you have chosen to take a new path using the Ketogenic diet plan. The plan is recognized by several names, including the low-carb diet, Ketogenic low-carbohydrate diet & high-fat (LCHF) diet plan, and the Keto diet.

Your liver produces ketones, which are used as energy to provide sufficient levels of protein. The process of ketosis is natural and occurs daily – no matter the total of carbs consumed.

Before you begin the journey to ketosis; here is a bit of insight on how the diet plan was discovered:

During history as early as the 20th century, fasting was theorized by Bernard McFadden/Bernarr Macfadden as a means for restoring your health. One of his students introduced a treatment for epilepsy using the same plan. In 1912, it was reported by the New York Medical Journal that the fast is a successful method to treat epileptic patients, followed by a starch- and sugar-free diet.

In 1921, Rollin Woodyatt noted the liver produced the ketone bodies (three water-soluble compounds, β-hydroxybutyrate, acetone, and acetoacetate) as a result of a diet low in carbohydrates and rich in fat.

Also, in 1921, Dr. Russell Wilder, who worked for the Mayo Clinic, became well-known when he formulated the keto plan, which was then used as part of the epilepsy therapy treatment plan. He had a considerable interest in the project because he also had epilepsy. The program became known for its other effects which helped in weight loss, and many other ailments.

The ketosis dieting technique was set aside in the 1940s because "improved" methods were discovered for the treatment of epilepsy. However, during that time - approximately 30% of the cases using the alternate plan failed. Therefore, the original

Ketogenic plan was reintroduced to the patients. As of 2016, Wilder is still functioning successfully without the seizure episodes.

As a direct result of Dr. Wilder's discovery, innovation began at the Mayo Clinic. Another physician standardized the diet plan using the following calculation:

- 10-15 carbs daily
- 1 gram of protein per kilogram of bodyweight
- The remainder of the count will remain with fat

As time passed, the plan had a few changes to make it functional as it is today.

The family of Charlie Abraham founded the Charlie Foundation in 1994 after his recovery from seizures he had daily, and other health issues. Charlie—as a youngster—was placed on the diet and continued to use it for five years. As of 2016, he is still functioning successfully without the seizure episodes and is furthering his education as a college student.

The Ketogenic diet has been utilized for 92 years as a weight loss diet and a means of controlling certain medical conditions. We are going to take a look at the basics of the Ketogenic diet to show how it can work for you today. The Ketogenic diet is a low carb diet that contains a moderate amount of protein, low carbohydrates, and high-fats. The Ketogenic plan focuses on reducing the percentage of carbs eaten to force the body to break down fats instead. The keto diet was made specifically for you to reach ketosis. Ketosis is a metabolic state where your body produces ketones. Ketones are provided by your liver and are used as fuel towards your body and brain instead of glucose. To make ketones, your diet must be low in carbs and only an adequate amount of protein. The Ketogenic diet is often compared to other foods like the Atkins diet and the Paleo diet.

While both the Atkins and Paleo diet's focus on cutting carbs down, there is a significant difference in how each plan uses this reduction in carbohydrates. The Ketogenic diet relies on deficient levels of carbohydrates to put the body into a state of ketosis throughout the entire menu. This enables your body to continue to rely on fat-burning rather than sugar (glucose) burning for energy. The Atkins diet relies upon a lack of carbohydrates in the initial phase of dieting but then reintroduces carbs gradually at lower rates. The paleo diet, however, can or cannot be Ketogenic because it does allow for the consumption of starches. Additionally, the paleo diet does not necessarily have to include higher levels of fats like the Atkin's, and Keto foods do.

One other way that the Ketogenic diet stands out from other diets is because it has a medical application for individuals with epilepsy. Research has shown that higher levels of ketones in the blood have been proven to reduce seizure activity. So the Ketogenic diet has applications for those with epilepsy or other seizure disorders. Usually, you get your energy from glucose, but on a Ketogenic diet, your body switches its fuel source to burning fat. When this occurs, your insulin levels will be low, and you will be burning fat always. Many people can safely follow a Ketogenic diet. Still, in some situations, you should take a more logical approach, for example, if you have diabetes, high blood pressure, or breastfeeding, you should research for alternatives. Since the Ketogenic diet changes the way that your body metabolizes nutrients. It is essential to check in regularly with your primary physician or dietitian.

Regular checks will help you to ensure that you are maintaining sufficient levels of nutrients and not pushing your body over the limits. It should be noted here that at ANY time you are considering a new diet plan, you MUST check in with your primary physician or dietitian! A quick check will make sure that a dietary plan like the Ketogenic diet is safe for you based on your current body mass as well as with any other existing health conditions.

Types of Ketogenic Diets

There are four main types of the Ketogenic diet, including:

Standard Ketogenic Diet (SKD): This is a very low-carb moderate-protein and high-fat type of diet. The standard food contains 75% of fats, 20% of protein, and only 5% of carbohydrates or less.

Cyclical Ketogenic Diet (CKD): This diet involves a period of high carb refeeds, for example, five days where you eat Ketogenic, followed by two days where you eat high carbs.

Targeted Ketogenic Diet (TKD): This diet is meant for athletes or those who exercise daily. It is where you eat mostly Ketogenic and high carbs during workouts.

High-Protein Ketogenic Diet: This is much like the standard Ketogenic diet; the only difference is that it includes more protein. The high-protein diet contains 60% fat, 35% protein, and only 5% of carbohydrates or less. Throughout this book, we will only be focusing on the standard Ketogenic diet. But if you hold much interest in the other Ketogenic diet versions, feels free to study them extensively.

Some Side Effects to Lookout For

Now the truth is, if you are not used to the Ketogenic diet, you might notice some side effects from it. Many people get demotivated after they follow this plan, simply because they don't feel like this plan will do them any good. However, let me assure you that these things will go away very quickly, so you don't have to worry about it. The first thing you will notice would be the keto flu. Many people who follow the Ketogenic diet tend to get sick in the first week. Which is fine, as it could be a part of the food. There is no explanation as to why people get sick within the first week, but it is something that happens. Make sure you take some time for recovery before you jump back on a diet. The second thing you might notice would be that throwing up would occur from time to time. This will only happen in the first few weeks, against freak out as many people experience this. The reason why an individual might throw up is simply that they are not accustomed to the high-fat diet. Keep that in mind, and if it makes you feel any better, have some carbs after you have thrown up. One of the significant side effects you might notice is nausea or even feeling like fainting if you feel like that, please make sure you have a look at your food consumption. Having an understanding of how much you are eating, especially on a Ketogenic diet, is very critical. Make sure that you are eating enough, as some people under eat when following the Ketogenic diet, overall, be cautious of this. Hunger is something you will notice when following the Ketogenic diet. Please note that the Ketogenic diet will only make you feel the excessive desire in the beginning once you get accustomed to the food it will go away. The last side effect you will notice would be bad breath. Please note that the bad breath will go away eventually. However, in the beginning, you will have a metallic smelling breath. Feel free to have some low-carb gum and water to combat this issue. Lemon water with no added sugar works the best if you can handle the sourness.

Chapter 2: Benefits of the Ketogenic Diet

The most apparent benefit of the Ketogenic diet is, of course, weight loss. While you will find that pretty much any food can help you lose weight if you cut enough calories, the Ketogenic diet is explicitly optimized for fat loss. If you've been struggling to shed a spare tire or you've wanted to whittle your waist, the Ketogenic diet may be just what you've been looking for. But how exactly does the Ketogenic diet work for weight loss? The concept is relatively simple. When you reduce your carbohydrate intake so that your body no longer has stored glucose to burn for fuel, it has to find something else to consume. In addition to burning the fat you eat, your body will also start to hack away at your stored fat. Numerous research studies have shown that the Ketogenic diet is much more effective in burning fat than low-fat and high-carb diets. The body needs fats as raw materials to produce ketones for fuel! In addition to increasing fat burn, the Ketogenic diet will also reduce insulin production, so you stop storing fat. That means that even if you do overeat once in a while, you're not going to undo all of the progress you've made with the diet. You will also find that the Ketogenic diet reduces your appetite, so you feel less hungry between meals, and that will help keep you from snacking and overeating. All of the above is fine and dandy and of course, great to hear, but what exactly is the science behind all these great benefits and more? Let's find out!

Natural Weight Loss

This is pretty much one of the main drivers for many, many folks taking up the Ketogenic diet, at least I know I was also one of them hopping on the bandwagon when I knew I needed weight loss in order to improve my health situation. The Ketogenic diet is really great for weight loss, as you will soon find out when you embark on the meal plans and really get into ketosis. The true magic of this is that you engage your body to help you out in losing the weight, instead of relying on calorie counting and restrictions to generate fat burn. When we first start out on the diet, we will begin to lose water weight in the initial stages. The reason for this is primarily due to our stored carbohydrates being present in mainly liquid glycogen form. As we reduce the reliance on carbohydrates, the body draws down upon these easily available stores of energy first as it grapples with the transition into ketosis. This water weight loss can account for anything from 5 to 20 pounds, depending on your initial starting weight when you begin the keto diet. This is a great morale booster to be sure, and most folks credit the keto diet with the lost weight. If we were to be very exacting in our specifications though, this water weight loss is actually due to us restricting our carbs rather than the actual process of fat-burning ketosis.

As we get beyond the first few days and transit into the first few weeks of being on the keto diet, that is when further drops on the weighing scale will definitely be recorded. The key here is the carbohydrate restriction that we have been constantly harping on. As a source of quick fuel, carbs can be second to none. The glucose obtained from the carbs channel quickly into all areas of the body and provide them with the necessary energy boost when needed. The downside for this is that our bodies aren't really built for storing carbs. We really cannot store beyond a day or two of energy unlike our fat stores. When we cut down on carbs, the body goes into ketosis as we all know by now. This nature's alternate plan for energy would see fats being processed through the liver and then converted into energy-giving ketones. That is also part of the reason why some folks actually term the Ketogenic diet as a starvation diet.

In a sense, they are not wrong, because this alternate way for the body to produce energy actually can sustain a human for up to a month without ingestion of food. The fat stores become the fuel for energy. However, I would definitely have to state most strongly that we are not starving ourselves whilst on the keto diet. Just because ketosis is nature's way of not letting us starve when we are deprived of food does not mean there should be any negative connotations attached to it. More importantly, whilst on the keto diet, we have to remember that we are not really counting calories and it is a definite must to eat when we feel hungry.

When our body successfully transits into burning fat for fuel, this would mean the stored fat as well as the fat that we consume daily would become fair game for ketone production. The trick here is the need to let the body get accustomed to burning fat instead of glucose, which is the main reason why the keto diet is a high-fat low carb diet. As long we do not break ourselves out of ketosis, the weight loss that we experience would definitely be from the fats, aside from the initial water weight loss mentioned earlier. No exercise, no calorie restriction, no weight pills and exotic berries which you need for losing weight. The Ketogenic diet simply enlists the body's natural functions in order to kick start this powerful process of natural fat loss, however this only works if you are obese workouts will be shown later. One thing to note however, this does not mean that you get to eat and binge all the way.

No matter what methods you use to lose weight, if you were to overeat and consume food even when you feel satiated, I would dare say it would be a tall order to instigate any weight loss if that were the case. Happily, there is something about the Ketogenic diet that also helps to prevent overeating. Read on!

Hunger Management

First off, when we wean ourselves from the carb-based diet and move on to a fat-based one, we are already doing ourselves a favor when it comes to hunger management. Carbs generally call to their own, like the sirens of yore that sailors in ancient times feared so much. Tell me if you have experienced this. You finish a bag of chips or perhaps three chocolate doughnuts, and within an hour or two, your stomach growls a little and there is that little, warmish feeling at the pit of your belly signaling that it is about time to find food again. The primary cause of this would be due to the blood sugar fluctuations happening whenever there is an over the top intake of glucose. We would be talking more about this in the later segment, but it would suffice now to say that when we transit to a primarily fat-based diet, this issue with the carbs meddling with the feelings of hunger will go away. As we move into ketosis and the body activates the fat-burning process for energy, we would generally feel less instances of hunger and more feelings of satiety. This occurs even if we were to be eating just two meals in a day, which I must say, is quite common amongst keto practitioners. As we take in more fat and moderate amounts of protein, these two essential macronutrients have the ability to let you feel satiated and get that feeling of fullness for longer periods of time than if you were on a carb-based diet.

Couple this with the fact that the majority of processed and unhealthy foods have plenty of carbs in them, it shouldn't come as too much of a surprise that you would start feeling less hunger as you cut out these empty calories and replace them with nutrient-dense whole foods consisting of fat and protein. Beyond this, being in ketosis actually causes a double whammy effect on the hormones that control hunger pangs. Ghrelin, the hormone that makes us feel hungry, sees its production being muted when our body is in ketosis. This is good news because ghrelin usually increases whenever we engage in any traditional dieting and start losing weight. This would mean that you would be stuck in between a rock and a hard place. The more you try to lose weight via conventional dieting, the more hunger you would feel due to increased ghrelin production! Besides this, the hormone that controls the feeling of satiety, cholecystokinin, experiences a complete reversal of what just happened to ghrelin whilst the body is deep in ketosis. Typically, as you lose weight, cholecystokinin production decreases in a bid to induce you to eat more. However, ketosis prevents the levels from dropping even when the body is experiencing weight loss.

This works out very well for anyone who is on the keto diet because we get spared the hunger pangs that usually accompany traditional dieting. Some have actually asked if this would mean that the body may potentially waste itself into nothingness since feelings of hunger are suppressed and we may not know if we are truly hungry. To answer this, we would first have to come to an understanding that the body, as an organism, is a wonderful, intricately balanced piece of self-learning machine. The ability for the body to sort itself out is virtually second to none. When we are in ketosis, we will still experience hunger as our energy stores run down through expenditure via daily activities. These feelings of hunger are what I would consider as true hunger, as they are not created from a carb induced state of affairs. When you feel such hunger on the Ketogenic diet, it is usually a very strong signal to get your next meal! At least that is what I always do. That is why many keto practitioners always talk about eating only when you truly feel hungry and not be subjected to the usual social norms of eating during breakfast, lunch and dinner times. It really can feel quite liberating to be in touch with your body's needs. So, the idea that we would gradually waste away to nothingness really does not hold much water because we still would get signals of hunger to prompt us to eat. What really happens is that we get these hunger pangs less frequently than if we were to be still on a carb-based diet. The adjustments in the produced levels of hunger controlling hormones do play their part, as do the satiating feeling of fats and proteins. There is also another reason for the less frequent hunger pangs. We simply are getting more energy from the fat-burning!

More Energy and Mental Clarity

I am quite sure that I am not alone in having the experience of feeling weariness or even fatigue just after a meal heavy in carbs. Just imagine having had a hearty meal, perhaps even topping it off with a nice, sugary dessert, and literally within the hour you find yourself nodding off, scarcely able to keep your eyes open despite your best efforts. I know my many instances of bruised thighs can attest to how hard I pinch myself trying to keep awake.

The thing here with this fatigue is that it can be easily avoided, if you were to cut down on carbs! When the body breaks down carbs for fuel, the glucose generated needs insulin to act as a mediator in order to be transported into the various organs and cells to be used as energy. That is primarily the reason why our pancreas jacks up our insulin production whenever we have a carb-heavy meal. The body knows that it needs to safely usher the blood sugar present in our bloodstream to be used as energy or to be converted and stored as fats. In cases where our bodies are fairly young and not metabolically damaged, the resulting insulin sensitivity is still high, and the pancreas is able to create just about the right amount of insulin to match the level of blood sugar present. However, as we age and damage our bodies metabolically through inattention and diet, our insulin sensitivity decreases, and this leads the pancreas to produce ever-increasing amounts of insulin in order to ferry the same amount of blood sugar. The poor pancreas realizes that the body's cells aren't responding like they are previously to insulin and hence increases its production as a way to normalize the situation. This then results in a swift reduction of glucose in the bloodstream which triggers the tiredness.

If we give in to the fatigue and quickly go to bed, you might realize that we often wake up with a roaring hunger, which is also coupled with a strange feeling of bloated-ness in the stomach. When there is low blood sugar in our bodies, the body triggers hunger signals in order to get additional fuel. The bloated feeling in the stomach though, is a result of food not being fully digested. If we think about it, a hearty lunch should let us feel satisfied all the way until dinner time in normal circumstances. Why is it that we get feelings of hunger and fatigue just a few hours after our last meal? The key lies in the fuel that powers our bodies. Glucose triggers the insulin response, which in turn has the potential to create the so-called sugar crash that causes the tiredness and accompanying hunger. Energy-based from sugar or glucose can be compared to a candle's light, flickering and winking, subject to the whims of the wind. When your body is energized by ketones however, this power source is akin to an electric bulb, shining bright steadily and consistently.

When our bodies burn fat, insulin is hardly called into action. This limits the sugar crash possibility. Also, as fat is easier to store and more readily available than glucose in our body, the ketones produced from fat can readily draw upon our body's fat stores. We get a stable source of fuel as a result, which then explains why we feel more energetic on the keto diet as compared to a regular one. Ketones also provide more bang for the proverbial buck as compared to glucose, as they burn cleaner metabolically. When you place a plentiful source of fuel and couple it with the fuel's better energy-giving capabilities, is it any wonder that you probably would feel like being able to handle all the work and house chores, and still have energy for that special project which you have always been wanting to embark on? The buck doesn't stop here though. You may think having increased energy from the keto diet is really a great benefit. How about getting improved mental clarity to boot? Say goodbye to those days of fuzzy headedness and times when you just cannot seem to concentrate and be ready to embrace life with razor-sharp mental alertness.

What really happens behind the scenes to account for the boosted mental acuity, is the effect of ketones on the brain. Our brain hangs on the balance of two major neurotransmitters, glutamate as well as gamma-aminobutyric acid or otherwise known as GABA. Glutamate serves as a stimulant and is usually associated with intelligent processes, like talking or thinking abstractly. Geniuses are found to have higher levels of glutamate. Too high a level, without the balancing effect of GABA, would result in over-stimulation of the brain. This is when seizures, strokes and generic neurodegeneration occurs. As it turns out, glutamate needs the presence of the calming GABA in order to head off the potentially debilitating effects of over-stimulation.

What ketones does for the brain is to provide a more efficient way for which glutamate is processed into GABA, which then leads to a neural environment that has fewer neurons firing all at the same time. This translates to a real-world effect of having better mental clarity and doing away with brain fog. The brain also appreciates ketones as a better fuel. While it has to be said that it does require some amount of glucose to maintain a healthy function, this amount of glucose can be easily provided for via the limited carbs we take in as well as the process of gluconeogenesis, which is the creation of glucose via proteins. The difference between glucose and ketones as fuel can be markedly attributed to their oxidative footprint. Glucose, in excess, induces far more oxidative stress than ketones. Factor in the fact that the brain is literally a glucose hog while we are off the keto diet, and you have a case where it is a matter of when, not if oxidative damage would harm the brain. With the presence of ketones however, this oxidative damage is somewhat curbed and sometimes even reversed, leading to postulations about the neuroprotective qualities of ketosis.

Boosted Brain Health with Keto

You might have encountered instances where you have read about how the Ketogenic diet was used since the 1920s to help treat folks with epilepsy. It has been shown to reduce the incidence of seizures without the need for medication. In fact, treatment of epilepsy through dieting has long been espoused by the ancient Greeks. Hippocrates, the famous physician, was one of the forerunners of this therapy where medicine played a decidedly secondary role. Various research and anecdotal evidence have pointed to the efficacy of the Ketogenic diet in reducing or even totally suppressing seizures, particular in cases of childhood epilepsy. Recent medical research has postulated that the reason for these apparent benefits is mainly due to the increased energy production in the hippocampus, brought on by the introduction of ketones as fuel for the brain.

The increased energy levels found in the brain were thought to contribute significantly to ensuring more stability in neuron activity. The research also showed that the Ketogenic diet actually improved the brain's oxidative stress resistance, which bodes really well for other neurodegenerative diseases like

Alzheimer's and Parkinson's. Alzheimer's disease has been dubbed the diabetes of the brain, because the brain cells become insulin resistant and hence aren't able to receive their required amount of glucose. This deprivation of blood sugar to a glucose hog like the brain essentially means that fuel for neural processes is lowered, sometimes too much, and it leads to neural system damage. This then paves the way for Alzheimer's to take root. With the brain fueled by ketones however, insulin resistance of the cells can effectively be remedied, because there is very little need for insulin without reliance on glucose as fuel. Ketones also seem to provide an added layer of protection against oxidative damage.

For diseases like Parkinson's and certain types of dementia, oxidative damage to the brain cells, coupled with a lowered neural energy production, are thought to be the main culprits in letting these diseases take hold. When your body is in ketosis however, these two damaging factors are put on hold due to the presence of ketones. Another thing to consider is the impact of the additional fat that the Ketogenic diet introduces on the brain. The brain is effectively made up of about sixty percent fat.

There are tons of more benefits, but this should give you an idea of what the Ketogenic diet could do for you.

Chapter 3: Side Effects and Do's and Dont's

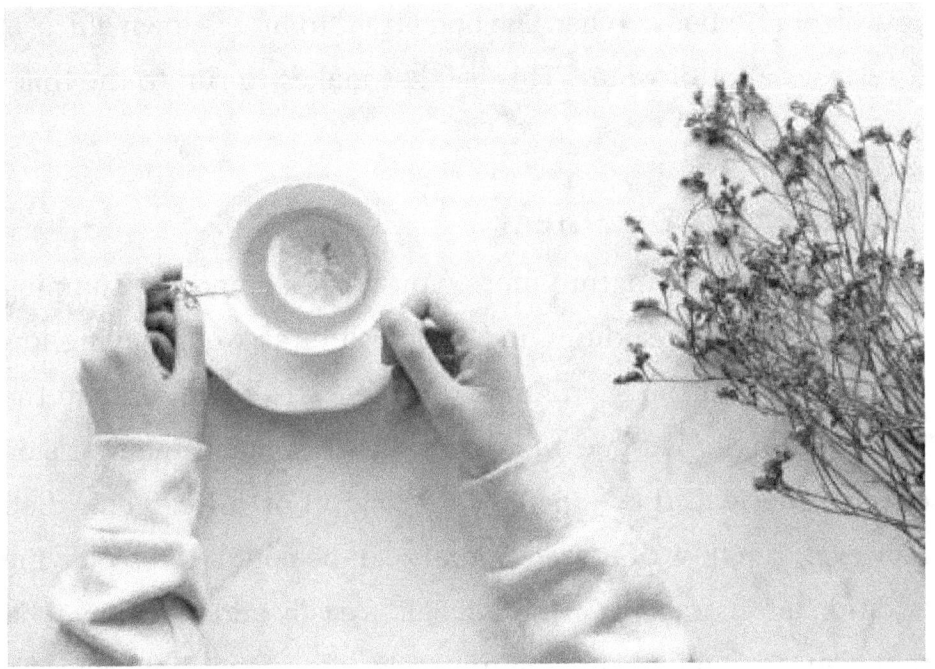

Now, you can easily understand why you are feeling the way you are after starting the diet and how you can control these side effects. What you really have to understand is that you are completely changing the way a normal body works and produces energy when you convert to a Ketogenic diet. It is quite normal for your body to resist and new change that you bring to it. But if you quit the gym on your first day because your body starts paining, chances are you are not going to go back to it any time soon. Some of the side effects that you may feel when you start a Ketogenic diet include the following. Urination After the first day or two, you will that you are being forced to go to the bathroom to urinate more often. This happens because your body is trying to burn the last bits of glucose that is stored in your liver and body. When the body tried to break down glucose, it releases a lot of water. This is what makes to run to the toilet more often.

Fatigue and Dizziness

When you start urinating more, you will also end up dumping minerals like salt, sodium and magnesium as well. Having low minerals in your body will make you feel weak and dizzy in the first week or so. Fatigue and dizziness are some of the first side effects experienced by a person starting off on a Ketogenic diet. However, the flow of these minerals can be countered by having additional minerals in your food. Salt is easily added on any food that you are taking and for minerals like potassium, you can have dairy food, vegetables and avocados. Low Blood Sugar Since your body might be used to getting high carbohydrate food before you transitioned to a Ketogenic diet, you might have bouts of Low Blood sugar. This is only natural, as your body is used to putting out insulin to counter the sugar that gets released by the intake of carbohydrates. This sudden change in your diet is what your body reacts to when you have low blood sugar. However, this will start to wear off when you are 2-3 weeks into the diet.

Constipation

Constipation is another common side effect of being on the Ketogenic diet. This is generally caused because of dehydration, loss of minerals, eating too much dairy or nuts or in some cases because of magnesium imbalances.

Sugar Cravings

As your body starts getting used to burning fats to fuel your body instead of sugar like it was used to earlier, you will start craving food with high carbohydrates. This is typical to last anywhere between 2-21 days. If you can fight the temptation, you will see that this craving will eventually start decreasing and then completely go away after a few weeks. It is essential that you do not consume any high carb food during this duration because it will stop the whole process ketosis. Diarrhea is another typical side effect of being on a low carb diet and it should go away naturally in a few days. This especially occurs if you start eating low fat along with low carbohydrates which results in a greater intake of protein. Ensure that you substitute the carbohydrates that you are cutting down on by increasing the intake of fats, preferably saturated fats like butter or coconut oil. To help you out of this issue, you can try to take a tbsp. of sugar-free Metamucil or plain psyllium husk powder before you eat a meal so that the fiber absorbs the excess water in the colon. This should help resolve any issue that you might have with diarrhea.

Shakiness or General Weakness

Both shakiness and general weakness are a side effect of low blood sugar, which sets in as you begin the Ketogenic diet. You can counter this by adding more protein to your diet and include foods that contain potassium. Alternatively, you can also take a 99mg supplement of potassium citrate. Sleep Deprivation People who are on a Ketogenic diet often complain about sleep deprivation. This may be because of low levels of insulin and serotonin in your system. To help with this, you can try to eat a snack which contains both protein and some carbohydrate right before bed. The insulin will increase with the intake of carbohydrate and this will enable more tryptophan from the protein to flow to your brain. This will in turn facilitate the production of serotonin which helps in having a calming effect on your brain. Another reason for losing sleep can be low histamine tolerance. Low carb diets are rich in histamine which makes some people anxious and deprived of sleep.

Kidney Stones

A lot of people who argue the use of the Ketogenic diet, sight this as a compelling example of why one must not follow this diet. This is generally based on the formation of kidney stones among children who are suffering from epilepsy. But that comparison is actually not very accurate. For starters, the diets given to epileptic children contain close to 90% fat and the shakes that are given to such children are made of processed powders like Ketocal. When you are on a Ketogenic diet based on real food, your body receives some amount of protein. Furthermore, there are reports to suggest that a dose of citrate supplement can deter this from happening among epileptic children as well. Low Thyroid Levels This side effect is also argued as one of the negatives of a Ketogenic diet. But that is only a natural response to a Ketogenic diet where your hunger is reduced. This same issue also arises when you are on a calorie-restricted diet made up of food rich in carbohydrates.

Racing Heart

A lot of people complain about having heart palpitations when they are in a Ketogenic diet for a few weeks or months. This is generally attributed to people with low blood pressure although there are several other factors that might be responsible too: This may be caused by the lack of nutrients in the system and can be stopped by the use of a multivitamin and magnesium supplement. It could also be that the person is resistant to insulin and the low carbohydrate diet results in hypoglycemia. Having homemade mineral water along with your breakfast and evening meal can help if this is the issue. Some people can have a racy heart because of the over-use of coconut oil and MCT (medium-chain triglyceride) oil. When you add these to your diet, it is advisable to first start with limited quantities and increase the intake over time. It is also advisable to not only rely on coconut oil and MCT oil as your fat source but also include other fatty foods like butter, ghee, olive oil as well as animal fats.

Even though a Ketogenic diet allows for some intake of protein, depending on the individual, it may not be enough for them and they might have to increase the protein intake. Increasing the intake of protein by 5-10 grams each day can help in such a case. Hair Loss There have been reports of people saying that they have experienced an increase in the amount of hair loss since they started a Ketogenic diet. However, this is natural in case of any change in diet and is not only restricted to a Ketogenic diet. This process of losing hair due to a change in metabolism or hormone levels is called "telogen effluvium." The lowering of insulin at the start of a Ketogenic diet is a normal but temporary side effect that could be a cause of hair loss among some people.

Low Carb Flu or Keto-Flu

As soon as you reduce the intake of carbohydrates to your body suddenly you start feeling all the symptoms of the flu – headaches, dizziness, crankiness and exhaustion. We have gone through these separately in the points above, but a combination of all these might feel to some people as if they have caught the flu, without really feeling sick. As soon as you start reducing the intake of carbs, you start feeling an urge to stuff yourself more carbohydrates. This is because of something known as metabolic flexibility.

This is a problem that some people might face only. Metabolic flexibility is a process through which your body can change its source of fuel from carbs to fats without any problem. If you, for example, have a potato with butter, your body will first breakdown the potato into glucose and use it power your body and when that is over, it will start breaking down the fat in the butter. But some people have impaired metabolic flexibility, which makes them cranky as soon as all the carbs in the body have been converted to glucose for energy. Their body instead of reverting to burn fats for energy, crave more carbs. If you eat a snack at this moment, your body will again use the carbs in the snack to power your body and all of the butter that you had eaten will get accumulated in the body as fats. It is almost certain that these flu-like symptoms will not last and will go away in a few weeks, but some of the things that you can do to fix this include: Take in the appropriate amount of carbs.

Do not shut them off permanently. Keep taking the amount that you calculated as per your lean body mass or ideal bodyweight. A lot of the symptoms are related to the drainage to the deficiency of minerals and salts in your body as you start a Ketogenic diet. You can get help on these my taking in more electrolytes. It is also important that you ensure that you are taking in enough fats as per your body mass index. It is impossible to run a human body only on proteins and if you keep insisting your body to use only protein as a primary source of energy, your body might just stop metabolizing and you will end up feeling starved even you have to intake enough calories. It is important to substitute the lowering of carbs by increasing the intake of fats in its place. A lot of studies have shown that exercise can help restore your metabolic flexibility but that can be a little hard to do when you are running out of steam 2 minutes into the exercise. If you can fight through the initial few days of these flu-like symptoms, you can start exercising after they are gone. Drinking plenty of water is extremely important when you are on a Ketogenic diet because when your body undergoes ketosis, it loses a lot of water and minerals initially. This causes dehydration which gives rise to headaches. It is important to note that not everyone who starts a Ketogenic diet goes through this "low-carb flu." In most cases, there could be separate incidents of headaches etc. that can be countered using the methods mentioned in the points above. Most people who are metabolically flexible will never even experience such problems. And even if it does, wait and be patient. This is only temporary and will eventually go away. As you can see, we have listed a number of side effects that people generally complain about when they start a Ketogenic diet. But most of these are only natural and can be countered by simple measures that have been documented in the points above. The ideal thing to do is, weather as much of these side effects as you can because they are all temporary and will generally go away after a few weeks.

As we have discussed many times over the course of this book, it is natural to find limitations in your body as soon as you start a Ketogenic diet. But as your body starts adapting to the use of fats as an energy source, you will see that your strength and endurance will soon start coming back to normal. The question to ask yourself is this: does carbohydrates enable us to build muscle? And the answer to that question is: No, it doesn't. It is still possible to refill the glycogen levels in your body when you are on the Ketogenic diet. The key to that is the amount of protein that you intake. If that part of the diet is taken care of, you can put on body mass even when you are on a low carb diet. What you can do if you are specifically looking to put on more body mass is that you increase the intake of protein by 1 to 1.2g per lean body mass. It is true that putting on body mass during the Ketogenic diet is slow, but it is only because the total fat content of your body is not increasing as it is getting burnt to provide energy.

People often misquote that the Ketogenic diet makes you lose performance. But reports suggest otherwise. A recently concluded test on trained cyclists who were on a low card diet for 4 weeks showed that they retained the same muscle mass as they did before they started the diet and there was no dip in aerobic endurance either. Over the course of the diet, their bodies adapted to the process of using fat as an energy source and limiting both glucose and glycogen stores. Another study conducted on 8 gymnasts also seemed to yield the same result. In the case of both the groups, they were fed green vegetables, proteins and very high-quality fats. So, this proves that even when you are doing long bouts of cardio, the Ketogenic diet will come across as a hindrance for you. An exception to this could be an exercise where you are required to do an exercise which needs explosive action. To boost your performance during such an exercise, you can help yourself to 25-50 grams of carbohydrates 30 minutes prior to starting the exercise. You can follow the following steps to know how to exercise when your body is in a state of Ketosis. Resistance training is a great way of building muscle as well shed fat and it does not require you to put in long hours at the gym to do so. You can try lifting in short but intense sessions to fasten the fat-burning in your body. It is advisable to train in shorter sets. The number of repetitions in sets should ideally be limited to 10 and repeated numerous times instead of continuing on for a long time. The short intervals in between the sets can be utilized by the body to build up any glycogen that it might have lost during the set.

Cardiovascular exercises are ideal exercised to perform when the body is in a state of Ketosis. Although a lot of people will advise against it, eating a small measure of carbohydrates after a workout session enables the sugar contained in the carbohydrate to travel directly to the muscles. If you find that you are not getting the desired results that you expected from your low-carb diet, it just might be that you are committing some of the common mistakes that people tend to make when on a Ketogenic diet.

Intake of Too Many Carbs

While this is one of the most common mistakes, this is generally the cause when you do not do proper research about how much carbohydrates are supposed to be enough according to your body mass index or ideal bodyweight. A lot of people think that anything under 100 grams per pound is enough for you to be able to produce enough ketone bodies to power your body. However, as we looked in an example before, with an ideal bodyweight of 150 pounds, ideally the most about of carbs that you should have is 30 grams only. Only when the carbohydrates are low enough will the body be able to switch from using carbs to power your body to using fats to power your body.

Intake of Too Much Protein

Protein is one of the most important micronutrients that the body needs to function optimally. Generally, having protein-rich food increases fat-burning. But, when someone is on a low carb diet, gorging on meat can end up increasing the intake of protein in your body. When the body consumes more protein than is required, the protein gets converted into glucose through a process called gluconeogenesis. This glucose gets broken down into sugar that gets used as fuel in your body instead of the fats. This breaks the ketosis state that the body is in. Too Little Intake of Fat A human body gets the greatest number of calories from the intake of foods rich in carbohydrates. If this source of calories is taken away, then the body will be starved of food to create energy out of. Some people, however, think that since having less carbohydrates is supposed to be good, so must be the case with having low fats as well. However, that is one of the biggest myths.

Without carbohydrates the body needs some source of nutrients to use as fuel and that is when it switches to burn fats into ketone bodies, which does not happen, if the number of fats being consumed is also low. If the carbohydrate and fat, both are taken in lesser amounts, the body will soon run out of energy and starve. As long as you are keeping away from trans-fats and from vegetable oils, there is no reason for you to be fearful of fats.

Low Sodium Levels

As soon as the body starts going into a state of ketosis, the insulin levels in the body start going down. One of many uses of insulin is it's able to signal the fat cells to store fat. And similarly, the kidney to retain sodium.

When you are in a Ketogenic diet, your body will start losing water and other minerals including sodium and this is one of the reasons many complain about dizziness, weakness etc. in the first few weeks of starting a Ketogenic diet. This is because sodium is one of the most important electrolytes that is required by the body for it to function optimally. The best way to work around this is by taking additional sodium in your food. One of the best sources of food is salt and increasing the intake of salt is one of the best ways of countering this shortage of sodium in the body. Impatience Another common mistake, which is very often repeated, is being impatient with the process of ketosis. By default, the body is designed to accept only carbohydrates as a source to fuel the body. So, if carbs are available to the body, it will always take preference over any other source as a form of energy. When you stop the intake of carbohydrates suddenly, the body needs to get used to burning fats for energy instead of carbs. And it might take a while for the body to primarily burn fat for powering the body. And during this period, as the body gets used to the new source of energy, it is very normal for the people undergoing this diet to feel dizzy or sick. Most people get alarmed as soon as they start feeling under the weather a little bit and resort to discontinuing the schedule and diet as planned earlier. It usually takes anywhere between 2-10 days for the body to completely adapt to this new mechanism of burning fats.

This requires you to be patient with yourself and trust the diet that you have planned for yourself.

Chapter 4: Ketogenic Diet for Younger People vs Older People

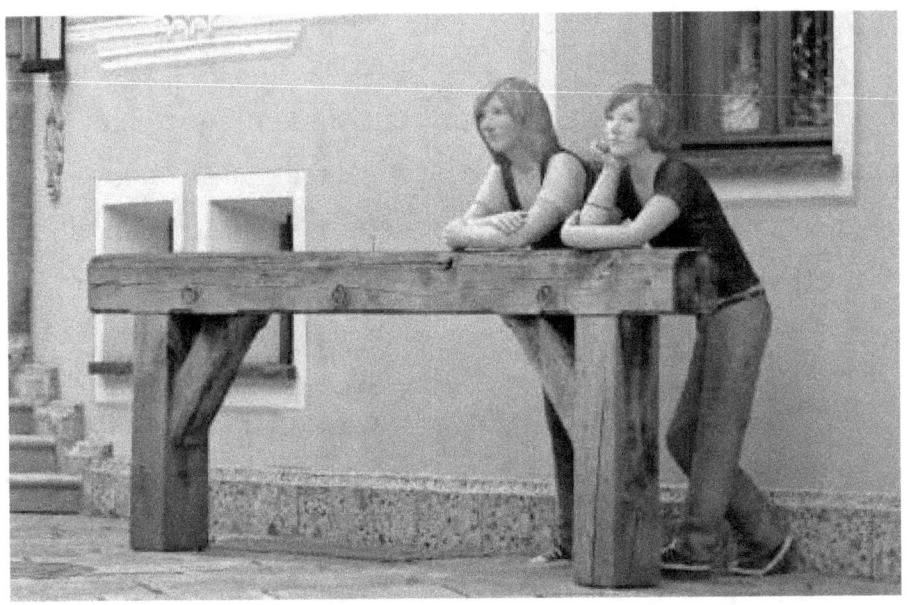

People think that is because it is complicated to follow in the beginning. We have explained to you what the Ketogenic diet is and what it can do for you. However, it is your job to understand how it affects your body. Time and time again, many people who are above the age of 50 have seen amazing results with the Ketogenic diet. The reason why they've seen such amazing results of the benefits, we have talked about the advantages which come along and Ketogenic diet, and they are very similar to the intermittent fasting benefits, which is why it is essential to understand that the Ketogenic diet can be a great asset to older people. Now don't get me wrong, the Ketogenic diet is for every age group and every sex. However, it is essential to understand the difference behind older people following the Ketogenic diet, whereas is the younger people following the Ketogenic diet.

The bottom line is that the Keto Diet is all about getting to ketosis, so for seniors this will present some unique challenges because they are not in the same physical realm as someone who is in their 20s and because of this, seniors need to think about the way that they do things, so that they can get the best possible results from the Keto Diet.

The good news is there are plenty of ways that seniors can use the Keto Diet and the process of ketosis to get some fantastic results. Actually, for seniors, there are many great benefits to ketosis, especially when it comes to keeping their minds sharp and their bodies active, so using the Keto Diet is something that will really invigorate many people who are seniors that are also healthy enough to take on the challenge of the diet. For seniors that miss the planning and the goal setting of working life, this is a great substitute because it engages so much more than the body.

There are many different things that come with old age, but just because you are getting older does not mean you should automatically be getting sicker. The bottom line is there is a connection between your aging and your health, and having a good diet is a great way to make sure that you are getting the most out of your senior years. In fact, when it comes to getting older, your diet is the easiest way for you to keep your vibrant and exciting lifestyle. As you age, there are several different ways that you can make sure that you are in optimal health. With that in mind, it is important to see the different things that ketosis brings to the life of seniors and how it is quite helpful. One of the things about aging that is impossible to reverse is the decline in our ability to do a variety of things.

We just simply are not able to run as fast as we once did, jump as high, and these physical limitations are something that is really impossible to reverse. That being said, if you are taking in a diet that has high carbs, all that you are doing is exacerbating the different problems that can be occurring within your body, so therefore, the Keto Diet is a great way to make sure that you are not putting yourself that much more behind the 8-ball. Getting older is not a reason to mourn, though, you can become a healthier and happier person and maintain a greater level of physical health as you age than when you were younger. This is why the Keto Diet is so popular with seniors. It provides many different ways for seniors to support their health and get a greater quality of life than they would if they followed the same diet from when they were decades younger.

This is perhaps the best part of being a senior on the Keto Diet – better health as you move forward. There are several different benefits that come with being healthy and staying in ketosis as you go ahead and embark upon this diet. Understanding these effects and how they can help you is a big reason why seniors will benefit greatly from the Keto Diet and being in ketosis. Resistance to Insulin Unfortunately, there are many senior citizens who are considered overweight or obese, and they are dealing with conditions that relate to insulin such as diabetes. The problem here is that diabetes can impair you in a ton of ways such as getting kidney disease, diabetic neuropathy, necrosis, and even things like vision loss. When you are in ketosis, this removes blood sugar from your system along with insulin, which is a great way to cut down on the effects of diabetes.

Bone Health

One thing that many seniors struggle with is the health of their bones. As seniors age, one of the biggest issues they deal with is osteoporosis, meaning that their bones become brittle. This is especially common among women and that means that a fall could end up being something that would be much more severe than it would have been just a few years earlier. The reality is that drinking more milk is not the healthiest thing to do, because lactose operates the way carbohydrates work in the bodies. There is a correlation too – countries that have the largest rates of osteoporosis are also countries that have the highest rate of dairy consumption. That being said, ketosis works in a different way. What it does is it prevents the body from having the absorption of nutrients that help blocked.

There are tons of micronutrients that go right to your bones instead of blasting them with calcium. These micronutrients fortify the bones and at the same time, keep you healthier than if you just were spending your time chugging milk every day. Healing Inflammation There are several ways that inflammation affects the life of seniors and nothing is more pronounced than the inflammation that occurs due to arthritis. The pain from these joint issues is something that restricts mobility and as your mobility is restricted, your quality of life will diminish very quickly. Getting rid of inflammation from a proper diet is much better for you than taking anti-inflammatories that can cause lots of problems with your kidneys and your liver.

The Keto Diet does a great job of naturally reducing the anti-inflammatories thanks to reducing the number of cytokines that are put in the body. When there are fewer cytokines, what will happen is that inflammation will lessen, and the joints will be looser and more mobile. Deficiencies with Specific Nutrients There are several different nutrients that people who are older have trouble with. The good news about ketosis is that it positively affects the different processes in your body. One of the first things that you need to rectify is iron deficiency. The problem with a lack of iron is that your brain will not be functioning all that well. You could get what is called brain fog and it is much easier to suffer from fatigue when you lack iron. Ketosis is something that will make sure that you get the right amount of iron so that your brain is operating at peak efficiency.

To that end, Vitamin B12 is something that is really important as well. Having high levels of Vitamin B12 helps prevent different debilitating neurological conditions like dementia. When you have high levels of Vitamin B12 this means that you will have a better chance of preventing the problems that come from Alzheimer's or Lewy Body Dementia all thanks to the Keto Diet. Fats are important to have as well – they make sure that you have great skin and vision along with keeping your vitamin levels high. Also, having the right amount of fats is important for making sure that you are having exceptional cognition as you get older. Vitamin D deficiency also causes problems with cognition as well, and it also increases the risk of heart disease and cancer. It has been proven that the Keto Diet and the process of ketosis increases the levels of Vitamin D in your system, which in turn means that the risk of these problems goes down. The idea that you could lower your risk of heart disease, cancer, and remain sharp is tied to your diet should be motivation enough to do the Keto Diet.

Finally, one thing that is easy to see and is a common threat is that animal protein that is found in the Keto Diet is a great source for all of these nutrients. The bottom line is that people can get exactly what they need from the Keto Diet, especially seniors. Closing these nutritional gaps is imperative to have a great quality of life. Regulating your Blood Sugar Levels This is a theme that has been hammered home many times already in this Book, but the bottom line is that your blood sugar is really critical to your quality of life. When you have unregulated blood sugar this is something that can cause problems with the risk of Alzheimer's and Parkinson's Disease. There are several risk factors that come with this.

For example, if you are excessively eating carbs that include fructose, you are basically daring your brain to develop neurological conditions. It has been proven that the Keto Diet and ketosis lowers your blood sugar, and that in turn lowers the risk that you have from getting these particular different neurological disorders. The insulin response of the body is something that has been talked about a lot, and when your blood sugar is out of control with diabetes, that means your insulin is not doing the job it needs to do. So, if you are on the Keto Diet this means your insulin is working the way it should and that your memory is something that will also be protected. Look, the worst stereotype about getting old is that your mind starts slipping. So, if you are in a position where you could change your diet and remain as sharp as ever, there is really no reason to avoid the Keto Diet. If anything, seniors should embrace it for this reason alone.

How the Keto Diet and Ketosis Is Important for Aging

The thing about the foods on the Keto Diet is that they deliver a ton of great nutrition and are packed with nutrients. If you have heard of superfoods, well, the Keto Diet is all about leveraging the food you eat for maximum benefit. The basal metabolic rate – also known as the minimum number of calories that are needed each day for survival – is less for seniors. But even though seniors need less calories than their younger counterparts, they do need the same amount of nutrients, and that is a place where the Keto Diet is of great assistance.

The reality is that people who are age 65 and older will not have an easy time living on junk food the way they could when they were younger. The body does not snap back the way it once did, and that is why seniors need to be more conscious about the food they are putting in their bodies. The food needs to support their health and fight disease. This is where the quality of life is found and where they can enjoy the years that they worked to get to. Why not spend them in enjoyment instead of being in pain and torment because your diet is compromising your ability to enjoy yourself. The reality is that seniors cannot have empty calories in their bodies from sugar and food that have anti-nutrients laden throughout them.

The reality is that fats and proteins that are rich in nutrients are what will make sure that people who are seniors can live their best life because the calories that they are taking in are being used by the body in the most efficient way and are not filler calories that would come from junk food. Furthermore, the food that is chosen by people who are older and are in different settings like a hospital or other clinical areas usually fairly brutal in terms of delivering the right amounts of nutrients. There is very little to gain from white bread, prunes, pasta, puddings, mashed potatoes, and other things that have lots of filler but little in the way of food that is actually good for you. The reality is that the government agencies that talk about the nutrition that you need are all about promoting a diet that is high in carbohydrates. The problem there is that this diet is not the one that is good for your long-term health. The reality for many people is that when they follow the standards that are published, they end up feeling less healthy and that in turn makes them feel worse for the wear.

This means that there is a greater level of cognitive decline and worse health. So, when going with the Keto Diet, what ends up happening is that ketosis helps people who are older get the nutrition that they need in order to make the most of their senior years instead of suffering through them and lamenting how they can't do what they did when they were younger. This is not how anyone intended to live in their retirement.

Using Ketosis to Achieve Longevity

The reality is that diet is a great way to improve your quality of life and when you are thinking about the rest of your life, do you want to live in comfort or to you want to enjoy what you are doing today for pain and discomfort in the future. The reality is we all should spend our time taking care of ourselves when we are younger so that we can enjoy the time when we are older. The bad news is that not everyone will use this high level of foresight. What they will do though is do the right thing with their bodies as they get older, and the Keto Diet is a great way to repair some of the damage that has been done over the years. The good news here is that making the changes that support a healthy weight, lower blood sugar levels, proper immune system health, and a high level of cognition will help get all the way to the optimal level of health. So, when you are a senior and you have a chance to really make the most of your golden years and all it takes is having a diet that is all about your needs, is there any reason why you would not take advantage of this diet.

Chapter 5: Ketogenic Diet and Working Out

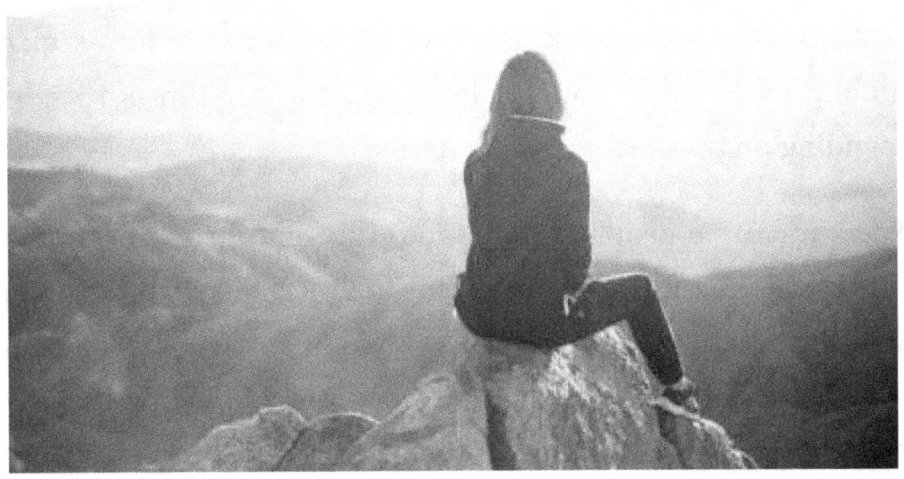

So, it's your first day at the gym, your goal is simply to get in shape and start living a better life. You walk into the gym, what the first thing you do is? Go lift in the squat rack? Maybe do some dumbbell/kettlebell work? Most likely, the first thing and the only thing that you would be doing is the treadmill or any piece of cardiovascular training. Don't get me wrong cardiovascular training is not bad by any means but in my opinion your primary focus in the gym should be on the resistance training, you don't really need a gym membership to jog/walk as you can go for a jog/walk even without the use of treadmill by simply stepping outside. I understand people who live in colder areas might not have the same privilege as someone living in a tropical area to go for a run outside year-round, but the point that I am trying to bring across is that your main focus walking into a gym should be on resistance training rather than cardiovascular training, but that doesn't mean you should neglect cardiovascular training either. Cardiovascular training needs to be done at least two to four times a week, depending on people's goals and needs.

I know for some people walking into the gym for the first time can be intimidating, you don't want to appear like you have no idea what you are doing here and be judged by fellow members and you certainly don't want to do exercises with weights because you are not sure about them. In order for you to get to your goals, you will have to go thru that learning curve which needs to be started the day you walk into the gym, Looking up instructions online on how to do these exercise is not that hard it barely takes any time to get the cue's and movement pattern down. The main key is to practice them, making sure you are using lighter weights and performing the exercise slower, so you feel the muscles that you are trying to work are indeed working.

If you do resistance training in this fashion for two to four weeks with three times a week of working out will teach your muscles to "fire" properly, and you will prime yourself to be doing exercises in a proper manner. Another way you can make sure you are doing your exercises right is by recording yourself performing it, then critiquing yourself based on the video you took performing that exercise. This method will give you a clear-cut idea of where your form is breaking down, and then you can go ahead and fix the issues that you are facing with that movement. If your form and technique are great, your risk of injury will go down significantly, and this is where you want to be at when you eventually get into more heavier weights, heavier meaning anything you will be performing for eight to ten reps and actually failing at the eight to ten rep range. I can't stress how important your first two weeks in the gym is before you start getting yourself into a program make sure you take two weeks or however long it takes to learn and perform exercises properly, but the main exercises you need to focus on are Pushing movement (push-ups), Pulling movement (Rowing movement), Hinging movement (deadlift), Squatting and Planks (core).

I will be talking about these five movements on how to perform them. These five movements are crucial and should be in everybody's training plan. Whether you are a twenty-year-old trying to get big or a fifty-year-old woman who is working out simply for health reasons. The first thing you should learn is these five movements, as these are the most difficult to learn and perform properly, but after you have managed to learn them, you will be in a lot better position to start incorporating other exercises. Now since you have gotten an idea as to how you should be starting with regards to resistance training, let's move on to Cardiovascular training.

The best way to start doing cardiovascular training, in my opinion, is just walking. Walking is one of the best methods for you to get started with its easy, and its really low intensity can also be really relaxing for some. Cardiovascular training should be done by everyone whether your goal is muscle gain or to lose body fat, no doing cardiovascular training won't make you lose muscle if done right it will actually help you recover from workouts, which will help you recover from the higher volume of training which will also help you put on more muscle in a shorter period of time. There are a lot of other ways of doing cardiovascular training we won't get into that in this book, as there will be another book simply on cardiovascular training on how to get the most out of it based on fat loss and other stuff.

Resistance Training is Key

I talked about how resistance training can be beneficial for anyone. Whether you want to put on muscle, lose fat, or just stay in shape, it is crucial that you have resistance training in your program. Now let us get into the specifics of what resistance training is and why you should be using it. Resistance training in layman's term is a form or a type of exercise that you use for muscular strength and endurance. Now let us get into the whys, and if your goal is to put on muscle, you need to achieve micro-tears in order for your muscles to grow stronger and bigger, this process is called hypertrophy. If your goal is to get in shape or lose weight having a greater amount of muscle fibers will raise your metabolism, which will help you burn more energy at rest, meaning fat and glycogen. If you're a fifty-year-old woman who just want to stay in shape resistance training will help you gain strength.

Now hypothetically speaking, if you tripped over and fall with no one around to help you get back up on your feet, you need strength to push yourself up off the floor, when your young that's the last thing you are worried about but as you get older something as easy as this could be a struggle. If you can't get yourself up off the floor and no one is there to help you. Guess what? You're in trouble, and the sooner you start working on your strength, the better. That doesn't mean you need to train like a bodybuilder. You just need to do some type of resistance training to stay at an optimal health level.

Now let's talk about resistance training for people looking to put on muscle, for someone who is trying to put on as much muscle as possible more volume is the key, usually, after a workout, people's recovery is about forty-eight to seventy-two hours. That is depending on stress, sleep, nutrition, genetics, but an average is forty-eight to seventy-two hours to recover from a workout. So, if you have gone online and looked up workout programs for bodybuilding, most of them are one to two body parts split, and you only train the muscle group once a week, that's a hundred and sixty-eight hours you have not trained that specific muscle. So, the conclusion is that you can train a certain muscle multiple times a week, which means you will put on more muscle and get stronger faster than someone who only trains that specific muscle once a week. Programming is going to be more than one body part a day, unlike a bodybuilding split, and will be repeated a couple of times a week for someone who has the time for it. Three to five times a week would be perfect for them to achieve their goals in terms of putting on muscle if not, then full-body workouts three times a week with higher intensity (heavier weights) can be used to yield similar effects. The main focus here is to train those muscles every two to four days making sure we are fully recovered first.

Now, for someone who is in their mid-fifties trying to get in shape because your doctor told you to or you have decided to embark on this journey yourself, then the resistance training part will be a lot more different for you than someone who is just trying to get bigger and muscular, our main focus for someone who wants to stay healthy and get in shape is to gain strength, start firing muscles that we have not used before and started putting on some muscle so we can actually achieve the first two things listed here. For people with the needs listed above, the best way to get to your goals will be full-body training meaning all your major muscles in one day, don't worry doesn't take longer than one hour to do so. You should perform these workouts three times in a week, main goal for this is to make sure we are using slow tempo meaning we are performing the exercise in a slow fashion and making sure we are actually firing the right muscle fiber, at first it would seem like it's hard to actually fire the exact muscles you are trying to fire. But if you consciously think about that muscle to "fire," eventually you will start to feel it, that is if your form is correct. Take your time with your technique first. Don't overlook it. That goes for anyone.

Sets, Repetition, Tempo

Let me explain to you what exactly, sets, repetition tempo is. Sets- how many times you perform an exercise before moving on to the next exercise. Repetition- How many times continuously you perform the exercises without any break. Tempo- How fast or slow you perform a rep. These three components are the single most important aspects of your training. You need to make sure you are actually following the rest set and tempo according to your training age, and your goals. If someone is in peak health and is an experienced trainee, then I would not make him wait five minutes before we get into our next set, Unless we are training heavy or going to attempt a one-rep max if that's the case then rest till we are fully recovered from going into the exercise.

Another thing that factors in when it comes to the three components is what your goals are and what type of training you are into or doing right now. If your goal is to get lean and build up your cardiovascular health, then shorter breaks with a fast tempo and with a couple of sets will work better for you to yield those results. Whereas we look at a different spectrum, if your goal is put on the most muscle as possible, then time under tension is the key, meaning that we will have to slow down the tempo and make the rest in between longer and do multiple sets of the exercise to yield those results. There is no cookie-cutter rest, sets, the tempo that will do for any type of workout. People who have been training for a while tend to need a lot less rest in between than someone who is just starting to work out, since it's a new stimulus for them.

Reading Tempo Breakdown

Now let me show you the breakdown and how tempo is to be read in a workout template. If someone writes for example 2:0:2:0 in a workout template, for example you are doing a push up this would mean that two seconds down would be the lowering portion of the eccentric, the second number would mean a pause at the bottom or in the middle the third would be the pushing up or the concentric portion of the repetition and the final would be at the top of the repetition, if there is a hole at the top or in the middle, it should be specified where the hold is in the middle or top/bottom. So this is how you would read how tempo is to be read. If the program has "x" in the tempo, it means lift as explosively in that lifting phase as you can.

Tempo Breakdown for Beginners

For someone who is just beginning to workout, slower on the eccentric (on the way down) and a little bit faster on the concentric (on the way up), the reason why is so that we can start firing the right muscle fibers because in the beginning stage of working out people tend to compensate other muscles fiber that they use most often. So, doing it slow something like 4:0:1:0 tempo would be a lot more beneficial for you.

How Sets Are Used for Different Goals

Sets are not so tricky as reps and tempo none the less still important that they are used correctly towards your goal. Now basic sets scheme is three sets, which can be used in a beginner/ intermediate lifter/ trainee who wants to put on some muscle. But if you're an advanced lifter, three sets might be the thing of the past. Let's talk about how sets should be used for a beginner who is stepping in the gym for the first time. 1-2 sets per exercise with a sufficient amount of break.

Do that for 2-4 weeks, depending on how you feel, and then you can slowly start doing two exercises in the same sets back to back. This will build more muscle endurance and give your muscles more time under tension. I would not recommend doing this if you are about to perform a really big compound movement like bench press, squat, or deadlift as the exercise itself is taxing enough, and if you back to back it will only make your sets moving on weaker, especially if you're training for strength. Then just focus on your major movements first, and then for your accessory movement back to back exercises can be done. If your goal is hypertrophy and you have been working towards the goal of putting on some muscle for about a year or so, then back to back sets can really be beneficial for someone who is training towards that. As it provides time under tension and you are able to add more exercises in your workout, which equals more volume, that's major when it comes to hypertrophy for bodybuilding. For someone trying to get strong higher sets and lower reps would be the way to go so higher intensity meaning heavier weights and lower reps.

Primal Movements

Most people workout because they want to put on muscle, or they want to lose some fat, and some just want to work out to get in shape and live a healthier life. All the scenarios above need to be doing something called a primal movement. These movements all together workout your whole body in such a manner that these movements will not only help you get stronger or give you that aesthetic look that you're going for, but this will also help you day to day life hence known as a primal movement. Normally there are four primal movements, but personally, with years of experience in this field, I have decided to make it five primal movements, so here they are 1.Squat 2.Inverted rows/Trx rows (either works and can be adjusted to your physical capacity) 3 Push-ups/ modified push-ups 4. Hinge/ modified deadlift 5. Planks/ Abdominal work (depending on your fitness level).

All these primal movements can be modified to be accessible for anyone with any fitness level. Let us just say you cannot do push-ups off the floor. What you can do to make this movement more accessible to you is by doing it off your knees meaning instead of your toes you can use your knees as a pivot point or use a bench or a squat rack with a barbell and have your torso more upright or in an elevation which will make it easier for you to perform a push up. That goes with any primal movement. All of them can be modified to fit your needs. If primal movements are getting easy for you, then we can also make it harder by adding some resistance and or elevating it. Making an exercise easier is what we call a regression and making an exercise harder is what we call progression. It doesn't matter if you are really advanced or just simply a beginner. Primal movements are to be performed to reach optimal results, whether it be you living a healthier life, or you simply want to add that extra pound of muscle. These movements are really powerful tools and should be used correctly for individual needs and should be done safely. Now I will go thru all the primal movements with you and teach you the regression and progressions to this exercise and go through that with you.

Squat Regression to Progression

Let's start with regression if you cannot perform a bodyweight squat; what you start with is something called a box squat. Simply squat back like you are sitting back onto a chair and then with one second pause onto the box get back up into a standing position, a proper squat would be when your knees and your hips are bellow 90 degrees when you look at it from the side, if that's hard for you to achieve even with a box then start with a higher box or chair sit back on it and get back up and repeat that for sets and reps until its starts to feel like a 5 out of 10 in terms of how difficult it is. Then to progress from that, do the same thing but lower the box or get a smaller chair. Keep doing that until you have managed to get below 90 degrees, now when going past 90 degrees on your box squats and it starts to feel easy then instead of pausing just tap the box and get back up instead of fully sitting on to the bench this will feel a lot harder, eventually when it starts to feel like a 5 out of 10 then you should be able to do bodyweight squats. If you can't, then regress back to box squats with the tap and keep doing that until it feels like a 3 out of 10 and then tries out bodyweight squats.

Now when bodyweight squats start to feel like a 5 out of 10, then we can slowly start using some resistance to make it more challenging for you, so one of the ways you can make this challenging is by performing something called a goblet squat basically what it is you hold a kettlebell or dumbbell, and you hold it up to your chest level with both of your hands, if this description doesn't explain the exercise properly there are a lot of videos online that will show you how to perform them in a detailed manner. If you don't have access to any kettlebell or dumbbell, then you can wear a backpack, and you load the backpack up with some heavier things lying around at your disposal, something like a heavy textbook or bottle of water. When you are capable of doing more than 45 lbs of kettlebell, dumbbell, or any weight form used on the squat for reps, then we can perhaps get into a safety bar squat or a barbell back squat which one you move to depends on your shoulder mobility.

Rowing/Pull-ups Regression to Progression

Rowing is pretty easy to regress and progress from, the first thing you can start with is band rows or machine rows. Whatever you have available to you start light and slowly up the resistance, whether it be bands or machine rows. When you have managed to row about 3/4 of your bodyweight for 10 reps using machine rows or bands then you should be able to do an inverted rows, if you are using bands as resistance but you don't know what's the resistance in pounds then get up to the heaviest band you have and row that for 10 and then try inverted rows you should be able to get it done, beware there as bands with insane resistance, so don't take banded rows lightly. When you are able to do inverted rows, you should be closer to doing a pull up if you can complete a full bodyweight pull up great; if not, here are a couple of things you can do. If you have a pull up assisted machine you can use that, start with a weight that you can do pull-ups with for 10 to 12 reps with and when it starts to feel like a 5 out of 10 then lower the weight, so you get less resistance then repeat the same process until you can do a pull up.

Let's say don't have access to Pull up assistance machine what you can do is use bands to make it easier for you, simply hang the band in the middle of the pull up bar or if you have a pull up bar with different grips then just hang it on to the handle that you aren't going to be using. Now from there simply get one of your knees onto the band and start doing pull-ups this will help you get some resistance from the band, which will make it easier for you to do a pull up, same principle applies as assisted pull up machine, go to a lighter band when it starts to feel like a 5 out of

10 at the end you should be able to do a pull up. Now let's just say you don't have access to bands or pull up assistance machine in that case you can do something known as eccentrics all you need to is simply get at the top of the pull up bar by using a chair or something elevated to get you to the top without any effort and from there slowly lower yourself and repeat the process, combine this with other back excises to strengthen your back and then you should be able to complete a pull up.

Push-Ups Regression to Progression

Same as rows push-ups should be easy to regress and progress from if you can't do a push up off the floor, here are a couple of things you can do to make it happen. If you have access to a squat rack and a barbell what you can do is simply do push-ups from an elevation meaning place the barbell on the latches that the squat rack has on them and then simply do push-ups from there so your torso is elevated which will make it easy for you to do push-ups, let's say you can do push-ups off number 13 on the squat rack riser keep doing that until it feels like a 5 out of 10 in terms of how hard it then lowers the latch and keep doing that until you can do a push up off the floor. Now let's just day you don't have access to a squat rack simply do push-ups off your knees and use that as your pivot point instead of your toes after when it feels like a 5 out of 10 then you should be able to do a push-up. If you can't even do push-ups off your knees, what you can do is do more exercises that strengthen shoulders, triceps, and chest and then try doing push-ups off your knees you should be able to eventually.

Hinge/Deadlift

The main thing in the deadlift/ hinge is not to squat the movement. Instead, hinge it. I see a lot of people do this movement incorrectly for a lot of reasons, their lower back is rounding, or they are squatting the weight instead of performing a deadlift, there are a lot of other faulty movement patterns that can be causing poor form in the deadlift/hinge, but we will cover the basics. What does it mean to hinge instead of squatting? Simply put, push your hips back. Believe it, or not a lot of people tend to have issues pushing their hips back and leaning your torso forward while keeping your back straight could be a lot of reasons, but one of them could be gluteus and hamstring tightness, which you should be working on in order to achieve a great deadlift/hinge.

Now since we have gotten that covered first exercise which will progress us to a proper deadlift is kettlebell/ dumbbell and will be using a riser or a stool to which you will be touching your kettlebell/ dumbbell to as you are leaning your torso forward and pushing your hips back, meaning that the stool will be behind you and low enough for you to bend your torso forward while keeping your back flat, depending on your fitness and mobility level adjust the height of the riser/stool.

So best cue for a deadlift/hinge would be:

1. Stand up straight with a kettlebell or dumbbell feet shoulder-width apart or slightly wider whatever you feel comfortable doing.

2. Bend your knees softly and have the pressure on the middle of your foot.

3. Push your hips back while keeping your arms as close your body as possible and keeping the elbows straight, not bent.

4. Touch the riser, which is behind you. Start off like that and slowly lower the riser height to the point where you are touching the kettlebell/ dumbbell off the floor while keeping your back flat making sure you are pushing your hips back instead of squatting, and if you have issues keeping your back flat and you can't seem to bring the level down of your riser while keeping your back flat it could be your gluteus and hamstrings are tight so look up some stretches on YouTube or google it and most of you should be able to progress to a lower riser or stool after that. After following the steps listed above, you should be ready to move into a Barbell/Trap bar deadlift.

Planks/Abdominal Work

Day 1

1. Push-Ups (based on your fitness level)

2-3 sets of 12 to 15 reps

Tempo- 4:0:2:0

Rest- 30 to 60 seconds

2. Hinge/deadlift (based on your fitness level)

2-3 sets of 12 to 15 reps

Tempo- 4:0:2:0

Rest- 30 to 60 seconds

3. Trx/inverted row (Based on your fitness level)

2-3 sets of 12 to 15 reps

Tempo- 4:0:2:0

Rest- 30 to 60 seconds

4. **Squats** (Based on your fitness level)

2-3 sets of 12 to 15 reps

Tempo- 4:0:2:0

Rest- 30 to 60 seconds

When you are performing the squats, push-ups, and rows, you are using a lot of your core as theses exercise require you to be stable throughout the movement, so in my opinion, a lot of core/Abdominal training is required, if you are performing abdominal exercises for aesthetic reasons planks might not be your go-to. Now let us keep it simple if you have a big gut, I would not recommend doing planks as it can put a lot of pressure on your lower back if you try and hold it for a longer period of time. When you perform push-ups you are working out your core, for someone with big gut push-ups is fine for plank substitute, I would recommend doing something like crunches or leg raises instead and do your primal movements, and when you have managed to reduce your gut, you can go ahead and perform some planks.

If you are on the chubbier side, you can do planks, but if you are on the side of being obese and your gut comes out alot, that's when you shouldn't be performing planks, just wanted to clear that out. Now let's talk about progression and regression, if you are starting off and you do have a bigger gut start off with leg raises/ crunches either works, I would recommend more doing leg raises as it is easier on your spine, but either works just to make sure your spine is flat as you can keep it on your way up, start with 5 - 10 reps when it starts to feel like a 5 - 10 add extra 5 more reps so on and so forth. Now for planks , start off with however long you can hold the plank for let's say 30 seconds, when the 30 seconds starts feeling like a 5-10 go up to 45 seconds keep doing this until you can hold a plank for 2 minutes, after than is achieved add more weight to you back to make it harder.

Resistance Training for General Population

I have noticed that most of the books these days that are based on fitness tend to be more advanced, by that what I mean is books will talk about how to deadlift and squat properly when they don't realize most of the readers need to learn the basics first, it's like trying to build a house with no foundation, guess what it will break with no foundation. Same thing with someone who starts of doing exercises like squats or deadlift with no foundation to support it. That's when perfecting primal movements come in to play in order to build foundation so you can eventually get into a proper deadlift without hurting yourself, so now you see the importance of training the right muscle fibers to get them to fire a certain way, so when you move into the primal movements you are ready to roll. That being said previously I went into full detail on primal movements and how to progress to a squat, deadlift and all the other primal movements I will make an example three day a week workout plan for you guys which you can follow to build a foundation and move into more of the advanced movements and workout plans and actually reap the benefits out of it instead of hurting yourself.

As always, with your knowledge, after reading this book, you can make your own workout routine and build that foundation. This Example workout is best suited for absolute beginners, although a lot of people who have been working out for some time can use it to get better results in a more advanced workout routine. This plan might look basic to some but trust me to do this or similar template using the knowledge you have acquired from this you will most likely not injure yourself when you move on to a more advanced workout routine and actually see more results from the more advanced plan you follow in future. The best way to follow this plan is one day on one day off rule, so if you do day one on Monday, then do day two on Wednesday and then day three on Friday. So, I highly recommend taking one day off between workouts, especially for "newbies." Although this book has been written by a certified trainer please perform all these exercises at your own risk as there is no professional eye to look at your form and technique, another thing there are couple of exercises that are in this example workout plan that I didn't go thru in-depth, please do a quick search online and you will find the right way to execute them.

Day 1.

1. Seated Band/ Machine row (Based on your fitness level)

2-3 sets of 10 - 12 reps

Tempo- 3:0:3:0

Rest- 45 to 70 seconds

2. Squats (Based on your fitness level)

2-3 sets of 10 - 12 reps

Tempo- 3:0:3:0

Rest- 45 to 70 seconds

3. Incline dumbbell press (use weights based on your fitness level)

2-3 sets of 10 - 12 reps

Tempo- 3:0:3:0

Rest- 45 to 70 seconds

4. Gluteus Bridges (Start with bodyweight and start adding resistance as you go along

2-3 sets of 10 - 12 reps

Tempo- 3:0:3:0

Rest- 45 to 70 seconds

5. Planks (Based on your fitness level)

Two sets of 10 - 60 seconds again based on your fitness level

Tempo- Just hold

Rest- 45 to 70 seconds

Day 2.

1. Squats (Based on your fitness level)

1-2 sets of 20 - 25 reps

Tempo- 2:0:1:0

Rest - As short as possible

2. Pull up/Trx or inverted row

3-4 sets of 10 to 12 reps

Tempo- 2:0:1:0

Rest - 60 to 90 seconds

3. Hinge/deadlift (based on your fitness level)

2-3 sets of 10 -12 reps

Tempo- 2:0:1:0

Rest - 60 to 90 seconds

4. Push-Ups (Based on your fitness level)

1-2 sets of 20 - 25 reps

Tempo- 2:0:1:0

Rest - As short as possible

5. Planks (Based on your fitness level

Two sets of 10 to 60 seconds again based on your fitness level

Tempo- Just hold

Rest - As short as possible

This workout format, with different variations of primal movements that I have pointed out, will yield you results for a lifetime — giving you better health and longevity when it comes to lifting weights and working out.

Chapter 6: How to Make This a Lifestyle

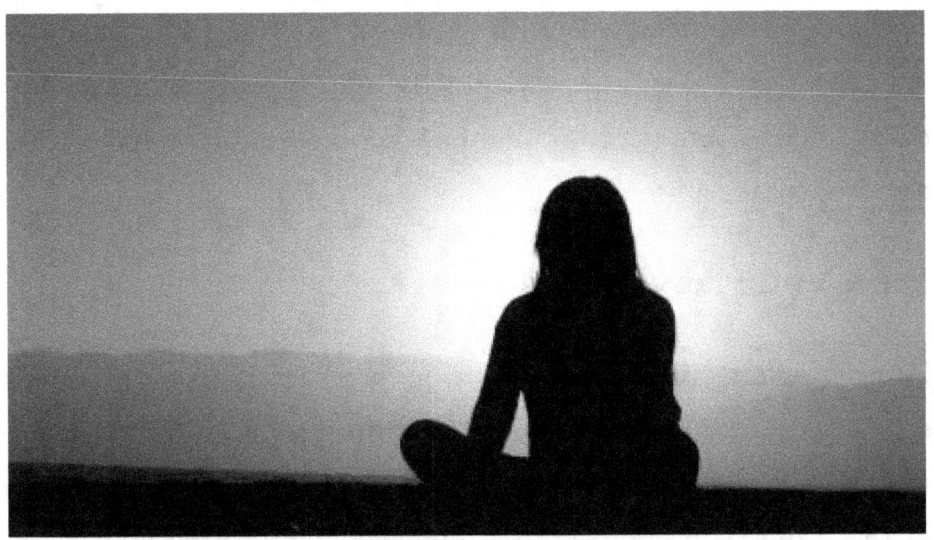

We will talk about what you should be doing, to make sure that you are not failing in your endeavors to start this diet to live a healthier life overall. This chapter will show you what you could be doing to make this diet your lifestyle and to not only help you to start the Ketogenic diet and stay on track but also to live with this eating plan for the rest of your life. These daily patterns will help you to not fail on your diet, and we understand that you might fail a couple of times in any diet, and it is understandable to do so. Nonetheless, this chapter will show you how to make sure you are consistent and not failing. These habits have been followed by many successful people, to get optimal results in all of their aspects of life, whether it be fitness related or anything else. Make sure you start implementing all of these habits after you are done reading this book as it will help you to make this diet your lifestyle. The reason why this chapter might sound philosophical is that the only way you will see success with this diet is if you do it consistently. For you to do that, you need to change your current lifestyle by being more productive and disciplined. You have to remember, healthy eating is more than just a meal, it's a lifestyle.

Plan Your Day Ahead

Planning your day ahead of time is crucial, not only does planning out your day help you be more prepared for your day moving forward, but it will also help you to become more aware of the things you shouldn't be doing, hence wasting your time. Moreover, planning your day will truly help you with making the most out of your time, that being said, we will talk about two things 1. Benefits of planning out your day 2. How to go about planning out your day. So, without further ado, let us dive into the benefits of planning out your day.

It Will Help You Prioritize

Yes, planning out your day will help you prioritize a lot of things in your day to day life. You can allow time limits to the things you want to work on the most to least, for example, if you're going to write your book and you are super serious about it. Then you need a specific time limit every day in which you work on a task wholeheartedly without any worries of other things until the time is up. Then you move on to the next job in line, so when you schedule out your whole day, and you give yourself time limits, then you can prioritize your entire day. The same thing goes for your diet, make sure you allocate time for prepping your meals for the next day, which will allow you to have meals ready for you when you need it hence making it easy for you to continue on with your diet.

More Focus on the Task in Hand

This point is quite similar to the previous point, once you have started to plan out your day and you have become more aware of the things that you are about to do. With the time limit on all tasks that you do daily, it will create an urgency to get as much of the job done as you can before time is up and you are moving on to your next appointment. Which will help you be more focused on the task at hand and get more things done? Many people consider healthy eating to be time-consuming, which it isn't if you prioritize your time the right way. If you cook your meals the day before and you set times for your meal, then it should not be a problem.

Work-Life Balance

You see, once you start planning out your whole day, you become more aware of your time and how to balance it out.

Once you begin to write out your entire day ahead, you will know precisely what you are doing that day, so you don't have to do anything sporadically throughout the day. Always plan some time for yourself every day where you can wind down read a good book, meditate or maybe hang out with your friends and wind down. You will feel refreshed the next day, having to wind down and "chill out" will only make you a more productive person.

Planning out your whole day ahead will not only help you prioritize better. It will also help you be more focused on your task in hand and will help you have a better work-life balance. This also means that you are eating foods that you like once in a while; this will help you to stay motivated with the diet that you are following. So now that we have covered the benefits of planning out your day, let's dive into the how to's when it comes to planning out your day.

Summarize Your Normal Day

Now, before we start getting into planning out your whole day ahead, you need to realize that to plan your entire day, you need to know precisely what you are doing that day. Which means you need to write down every single thing you do on a typical day and write down the time you start and end, it needs to be detailed in terms of how long does it take for your transportation to get to work, etc.

Now after you have figured out your whole day, you can decide how to prioritize your day moving on could be cutting out a task that you don't require or shortening your time for a job that doesn't need that much time. After you have your priorities for the day, you can add pleasurable tasks into your day like hanging out with your friends, etc.

Arrange Your Day

It is crucial that you arrange your day correctly, so the best way to organize your day is to make sure you get all your essential stuff done earlier in the day when your mind is fresh. After that's done, you can have some time for yourself to relax and do whatever it is that you want. But make sure you get all the things that need to be done before you can move on to free time for yourself. Another thing that will help you is to set time limits on each task, and once you start setting time limits, you will be more likely to get the job done.

Remove All the Fluff

So, what I mean by that is remove all the things that are holding you back from achieving your goals. Make sure you remove all of the things that are holding you back from getting the things that you need to be doing. If you have time for the fluff, do it if not, then work on your priorities first. In conclusion, planning out your day will help you tremendously! Make sure you plan out your day every day to ensure successful and accomplished days.

Be Grateful

We will be talking about how to be grateful and what are the benefits of being thankful for what you have! Now believe it or not being grateful every day will help you get more things done while keeping your mood elevated, see when your thankful for the things you have you will start to feel like your mind will be in peace and joy. When your mind is in order and comfort, you will be more productive with all the tasks ahead of you that day. Being in a grateful state of mind will help you become less stressed and more positive, which will help your work quality by ten folds. So, it is pretty essential that you stay grateful not only for better work performance but to also be in a peaceful state of mind. This will also help you to do more positive things with your diet, such as eat clean through the day. Let's discuss the three main benefits of being thankful.

1. **Helps you start your day**

Of course, if you start your day in a happy mood, you will more likely be keen to do more stuff and be more productive. If you read up on the most dedicated peoples and their day to day life, you will know that successful people tend to practice the same habits which I am going to be talking about in this chapter. The benefit of saying things you are grateful for, first thing in the morning will boost your positive vibes when you talk about the things, you're thankful for you will complain a lot less and attract negative vibes which is something we don't want! You always want to be in a positive mood as much as you can. To make sure you are in a positive vibe, write or say things you are grateful towards.

2. You will become more approachable

Yes, being grateful will make you more approachable! Believe it or not, people do sense your "vibes" when you walk into the door. When you're more thankful for life, you are happier and more positive, which is what people want to be around. Who knows the next person you see could be an opportunity for you to grow your business or get a new job! So always make sure you are in a great mood and counting your blessings still, as good things will come to you.

3. Lowered stress levels

I think this point is very self-explanatory, let me ask you this what most people are stressed about? Lack of resources plain and straightforward. A lack of resources creates 99% of the stress. Once you start counting what you have rather than what you don't have, you begin to become a lot less stressed, which is suitable for your physical and mental health! So, make sure you always stay in a grateful mood. If you want to understand more about how being grateful can change your life, I recommend reading "The Magic" by Rhonda Byrne.

So, all in all, being grateful will help you live a better life and be more successful. Now you might be wondering how to be thankful throughout the day since it is so hard to block out ungrateful thoughts, well I'll show you three techniques that will help you combat your ungrateful thoughts and keep you in a grateful "vibe" most of your life.

Write ten things you are grateful for every morning:

You see, writing what you are thankful for will make your life a lot easier and help you start your day in gratitude. What I want you to do is first get a notebook/diary, then as soon as you wake up, I want you to write ten things you're grateful for. This could be anything from small as having water to drink to have a nice car, the whole point of this is to make you start your day in gratitude as the way you start your day is the way your entire day is going to be most of the time. So, make sure to start your day on the right foot by writing down ten things you're grateful towards.

Don't forget the 1:5 ratio:

This is something I came up with, and it works great for me, you see whenever I say something I am angry or not grateful for I always say five things I am super thankful for right after to get myself into the grateful "vibe" in the beginning this method will be your best friend as it will save you from killing your "vibe."

Cut out negative people:

This task might be the hardest to do, but it is quite essential, see the people who you are around are the people who will create your personality. So if you are around negative people, you will develop adverse circumstances for yourself, so if you are around people who are not upbeat about life and find everything wrong and never see the good in anyone, you need to cut them out and be around people who are happy and ready for what life has to offer. Now I get it, some cynical people can be your family members, and you can't cut them out, the best thing to do is 1. Make them understand what they are doing wrong 2. Show them how they can change their life. And if they still want to remain the same, then keep your distance.

In conclusion, it is essential that you are in a grateful "vibe" as it will not only help you with your mental and physical health, but it will also help you attract better people and better circumstances. Don't forget to practice the three methods we discussed in this chapter for you to be in a grateful 'vibe" throughout the day and life! That being said I hope this chapter shed some light on the importance of being grateful and how it can make or break your life, and I hope you don't take this chapter lightly being grateful is the most critical thing you can do to turn your life around. So be thankful!

Now that we have covered the part of being grateful, and how it can help you with your day to day life and eating habits. Let us give you some concrete ideas on how to change the way you live your experience and to make it better.

Stop Multitasking

I think we are all guilty of this at a time, and if you are multitasking right now, I need you to stop. Now multitasking could be a lot of things, it could be as small as cooking and texting at the same time, or it could be as big as working on two projects at the same time. Studies are showing how multitasking can reduce your quality of work, which something you don't want to do if your goal is to get the best result out of the thing that you are doing. That being said, there are a lot more reasons as to why you shouldn't be multitasking, so without further ado, let's dive into the primary reasons why multitasking can be harmful.

You're not as productive.

Believe it or not, you tend to be a lot less productive when you are multitasking. When you go from one project to another or anything else for that matter, you don't put all your effort into your work. You are always worried about the project that you will be moving into next. So, moving back and forth from one project to another will definitely affect your productivity if you want to get the most out of your work you need to be focused on one thing at a time and make sure you get it done to the best of your abilities. Plus, you are more likely to make mistakes, which will not help you work to the best of your ability.

You become slower at your work.

When you are multitasking, chances are you will end up being slower at completing your projects. You would be in a better position if you were to focus on one project at a time instead of going back and forth, which of course helps you complete them faster. So, the thing that enables you to be faster at your projects when you're not multitasking is the mindset, we often don't realize how much mindset comes into play. When you are going back and forth from one project to another, you are in a different mental state going into another project which takes time to build and break. So, by the time you have managed to get into the mindset of project A you are already moving into project B, it is always best that you devote your time and energy one project at a time if you want it to doe did an at a faster pace.

It affects your creativity.

This is a significant disadvantage of multitasking, and studies are showing that multitasking can negatively affect your creativity. When something requires too much focus from your end, it becomes harmful to your creativity, and you need a lot more attention when multitasking compared to working on one thing at a time. If you want to succeed and live a better life, then you need to be creative, so if multitasking affects your creativity, then you need to stop doing that.

By now, you can see how multitasking can hinder the ability for you to work at your best. These three things listed above are a no-no when it comes to living a better and more productive life; not only does multitasking help not be prolific but makes you slower and less creative. So, all the benefits you thought you were getting multitasking was not accurate after all, nonetheless, by now, you might be wondering how to go about working most efficiently. Well, the best way to put it is to work on one project at a time, I want you to put all your time and energy in the project you are doing currently and not worry about other projects. Make sure you set yourself goals when you start the project which will help you be more efficient and faster at your work, so an example would be "you will not move on to another project until project A has been completed" or you have managed to hit a certain threshold at that specific project. So, to sum it all up.

- Do one project at a time

- Don't move on until it is completed, or you have managed to hit a certain threshold

- Set yourself a goal (time, quality, etc.)

All in all, multitasking will do you no good. It will only make you slower at your work and make you less productive. Making sure you stop multitasking is essential, as it will only help you live a better life. One thing to remember from this chapter is to put all your energy at one thing at a time, and this will yield you a lot of better projects or anything that you are working towards to be great. If you want to be more successful and live a better life, you need to make sure your projects are quality as I can't stress this point enough. You are probably reading this book because you want to get better at living your life or achieve goals that you just haven't yet, one of the reasons why you are not living the life that you want or haven't reached your goal could be a lot of things but, one of the items could be the quality of your work which could be taking a hit because of you multitasking. So, review yourself, and find out why you haven't achieved your goal and why you are not living the life that you want.

Then if you happen to stumble upon multitasking being the limiting factor or the quality of your work, I want you to stop multitasking and start working on one project at a time while giving it your full attention. What you will notice is that your work will have a higher quality and will be completed in a quicker amount of time following the steps listed above, which will change your life and help you achieve your life goals in a better more efficient way.

After reading this chapter, many might be thinking that this is more of a self-help book than it is a diet book. The truth is that we want you to understand how to live a better life by changing the habits that you are currently following. Truth be told, following a diet and making it a lifestyle is a lot more work than you think it is. For you to make it easy, you need to understand that you need to change your habits in order to be successful at this diet, which means you need to change the way you move the way you think and the way you perform. This chapter gives you a clear idea on how to start living a better life by changing up your habits, once you do change your practices you will notice that following the Ketogenic diet as a whole will be very easy for you. The reason why it will be straightforward for you is that you will change the way you move and change the way you live your life in general. Changing the way you live your life will not only help you get better results, but it will also help you to follow this diet as a lifestyle, many people confuse diet as not being a part of a lifestyle, and it is something that they're supporting to better their health. But the truth is that when they're following a diet, they don't realize that it needs to be a lifestyle for it to be a health benefit, if you want to be healthier then you need to make sure that you're taking care of your health 24/7 365 days a year.

This means you need to make this a lifestyle, and for you to make this a lifestyle, we need to understand some self-help techniques to keep it sustained for a more extended period. This is why this chapter is more self-help oriented, we wanted to make sure that this book is different than any other books that you've read when it comes to following the Ketogenic diet. The way we're going to be delivering it is by showing you how to change your lifestyle for the better instead of the worst. We're not just going to give you foods to eat and how to follow the Ketogenic diet, but in fact, we're going to change the way you eat overall and to make it a better experience for you once you start getting into this diet. With that being said, I hope this chapter was helpful to you, and we will see you in the next chapter.

Chapter 7: 10-Day Eating Plan + Recipes

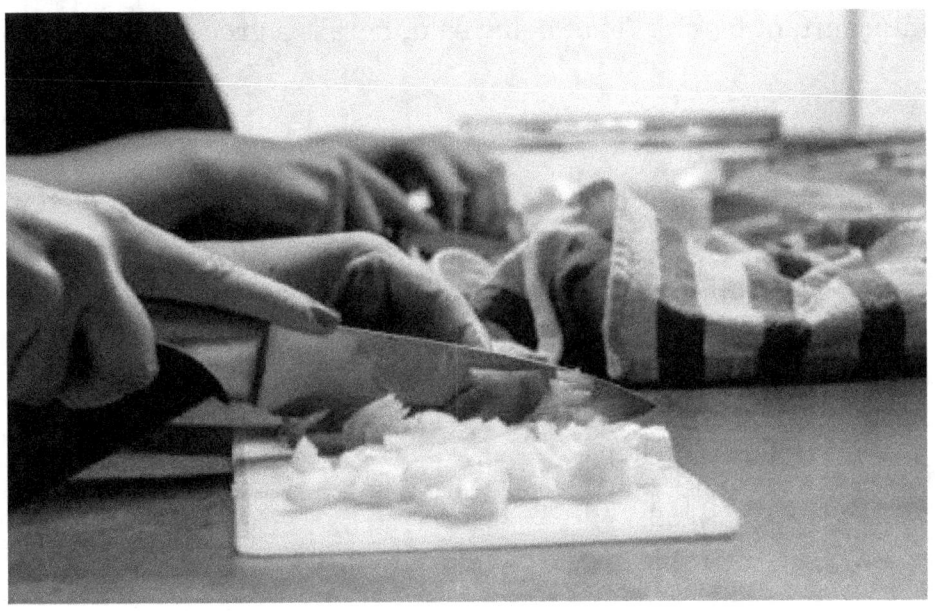

In this chapter, we will give you an excellent method to get you started. We will provide you with some of the most practical information you have ever used. Not only that, but we will also help you understand how to make a Ketogenic diet your lifestyle within ten days. Now, two things to remember when it comes to making the Ketogenic diet your lifestyle. Besides the fantastic recipes coming your way, you also need to have a great grocery list. We will give you the grocery list. Secondly you need to have a basic understanding of macronutrients. One thing you need to remember, would be that you will have to be in a caloric deficit regardless of what you think. If your goal is to lose weight, then you need to be in a caloric deficit. The only time you could get away with eating a little bit more would be when you follow intermittent fasting. That being said, here is a grocery list.

Things you need

1. Nuts (almond, cashews, peanuts)
2. Eggs
3. Meat (steak, pork)
4. Poultry (chicken)
5. Fatty fish (salmon etc.)
6. Low carb spices

You can always use the recipes for reference. However, these are just an essential grocery list for your Ketogenic diet. This will allow you to start having fun with the Ketogenic diet and seeing the results.

Now, the great thing about the Ketogenic diet would be that there is no requirement of you eating six meals a day. You can quickly get away with eating only three meals a day. Let us give you an eating plan to follow.

Breakfast: One of the breakfast recipes from the book

Lunch: One of the lunch recipes from the book

Snack: Handful of almonds

Dinner: One of the recipes dinner recipes from the book

This plan should be followed for ten days for you to see results. Two things to remember, the first thing would be that you need to count your macros, which is why we have provided you with macros on each meal. Secondly, make sure that you fight through the first ten days. This would be when the side effects subside. Now with that being made manifest, let us give you some fantastic recipes which you can start following today to see better results in your health and wellness. Please make sure that you use these recipes in your diet, as they will help you to be more successful in your keto goals. The great thing about this plan would be the tasty meals you will get to have. You will forget that you are following the Ketogenic diet.

Breakfast

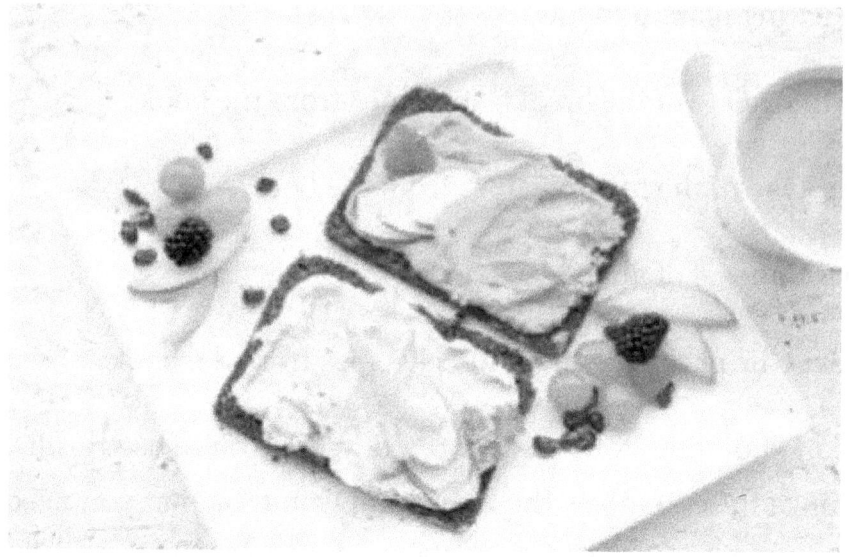

Almond–Chia & Coconut Pudding

Prep & Cook Time: 20 min.

Yields: 4 Servings

Nutrition Values: Calories: 130 | Fat: 12 g | Protein: 14 g |Net Carbs: 1.5 g

Ingredients:

- ¼ c. shredded coconut
- ½ c. of each:
  - Chopped almonds
  - Chia seeds
- 2 c. almond milk

Preparation Method:

1. Measure out all of the fixings and add to the Instant Pot, stirring well.
2. Secure the lid and select the high setting (2-5 minutes) Quick release the pressure and place the pudding into four serving glasses.

Deviled Egg Salad

Prep & Cook Time: 30 min.

Yields: 5 Servings

Nutrition Values: Calories: 313 | Fat: 26.4 g | Protein: 16.4 g | Net Carbs: 1.3 g

Ingredients:

- 5 raw bacon strips
- 10 large eggs
- 2 tbsp. mayo
- 1 t. Dijon mustard
- 1 stalk green onion

- ¼ t. smoked paprika

- Pepper & Salt to taste

- Also Needed: 6-7-inch cake pan

Preparation Method:

1. Grease all sides of the pan that will sit inside of the pot on the trivet. Pour one cup of cold water in the bottom of the Instant Pot and add the steam rack.
2. Crack the eggs open in the pan (try not to break the yolks).
3. Place the pan on the rack. Secure the lid and set the timer for 6 minutes (high-pressure). Natural release the pressure and remove the pan.
4. Dab away any moisture. Flip the pan on a cutting board for the egg loaf to release. Chop and add to a mixing dish.
5. Clean the Instant Pot bowl and choose the sauté function (medium heat). Prepare the bacon until crispy.
6. Add to the chopped eggs with the mustard, mayo, paprika, pepper, and salt. Toss and garnish with green onion.
7. Serve the way you like it!

Egg Cups & Cheese

Prep & Cook Time: 15 min.

Yields: 4 Servings

Nutrition Values: Calories: 115 | Fat: 9 g | Protein: 9 g | Net Carbs: 2 g

Ingredients:

- 4 eggs
- ½ c. sharp shredded cheddar cheese
- 1 c. diced veggies—example, tomatoes, mushrooms, etc.
- ¼ c. Half & Half
- Pepper & Salt to taste
- 2 tbsp. cilantro—chopped

Ingredients for the Topping:

- ½ c. shredded cheese your choice

Also Needed:

- 4 wide-mouthed jars
- 2 c. water

Preparation Method:

1. Whisk the veggies, eggs, Half & Half, salt, pepper, cheese, and cilantro.
2. Combine the mixture into each of the jars. Secure the lids (not too tight) to keep water from getting into the egg mix.
3. Arrange the trivet in the Instant Pot and add the water. Arrange the jars on the trivet and set the timer for 5 minutes (high pressure). When done, quick release the pressure, and top with the rest of the cheese (½ cup).
4. Broil if you like for 2-3 minutes until the cheese is browned to your liking.

Ketogenic Eggs

Prep & Cook Time: 20 min.

Yields: 4 Servings

Nutrition Values: Fat: 14.4 g | Protein: 7.3 g | Net Carbs: 8.3 g

Ingredients:

- 1 tbsp. chopped shallot
- 3 tbsp. ghee
- 1 sliced jalapeno—matchstick
- 1 t. of each:
  - Ground cinnamon
  - Cumin seeds
- 3 sliced garlic cloves
- 1 coarsely chopped green bell pepper
- 2 coarsely chopped tomatoes
- ½ t. of each:

- o Turmeric
- o Ground ginger
- o Salt

- ½ c. chopped cilantro

- 4 eggs—beaten

Preparation Method:

1. Add the ghee to the Instant Pot. Melt using the sauté function and add the cumin seeds, cooking until aromatic.
2. Continue cooking for 3 minutes along with the shallots. Stir in the peppers, tomatoes, jalapenos, and garlic. Sauté 3 additional minutes and add the salt, ginger, salt, and turmeric.
3. Whisk in the eggs and cook until set (30 seconds). When the eggs are at the right texture, sprinkle with the pepper, salt, and cilantro.
4. Secure the lid and prepare for 13 minutes. Quick release the steam and serve.

Lunch

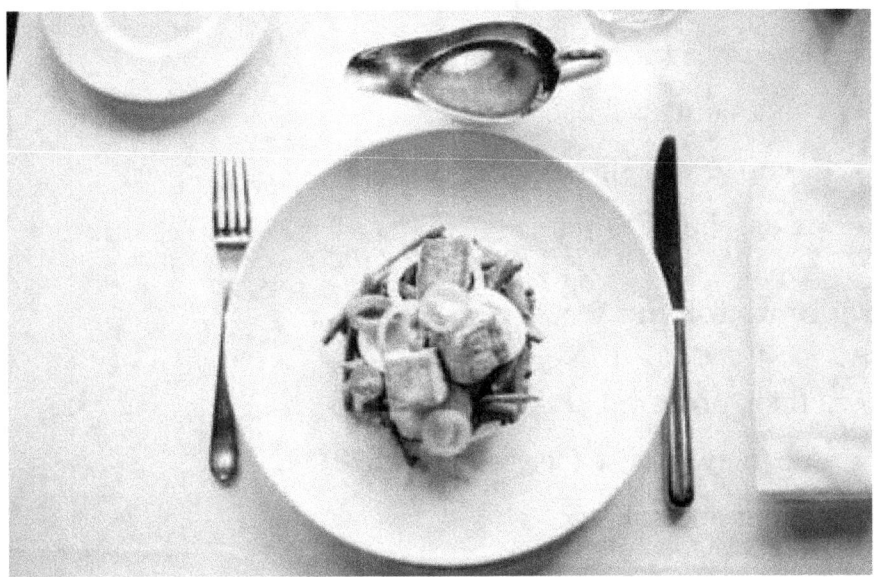

Salads

Bistro Steak Salad with Horseradish Dressing

Serves: 2

Nutritional Values Per Serving:

Calories: 736 | Protein: 41.4 g | Carbohydrates: 6.2 g| Fat: 59.4 g

Ingredients:

- 1 (12 oz.) rib-eye steak
- ¼ t. of each:
- Pepper

- Salt
- 1 (2.1 oz.) small red onion
- 1 (7 oz.) bag romaine salad greens
- 4 slices uncured bacon
- ½ cup (2 oz.) sliced radishes
- 4.2 oz. cherry tomatoes

Ingredients for the Dressing:

- 2 tbsp. prepared horseradish
- ¼ c. mayonnaise (see recipe below)
- Pepper and salt

Method:

1. Thinly slice the onion and radishes.
2. Place parchment paper on a baking tin. Set the oven temperature to 350°F. Arrange the bacon in a single layer in the pan. Bake for 15 minutes. Drain and break into small pieces.
3. Pat the steak with paper towels. Season with the pepper and salt. Grill for four minutes and flip. Continue cooking another 12-15 minutes (medium is approximately 12 minutes or internal temperature of 155°F.).
4. Let it cool down five minutes, and slice against the grain into small slices.
5. Prepare the dressing (below) and enjoy.

Low-Carb Mayonnaise for the Horseradish Dressing

Serves: 4

Nutritional Values Per Serving: Included with above recipe

Ingredients:

- 1 egg yolk
- 1-2 t. white vinegar/lemon juice
- 1 tbsp. Dijon mustard
- 1 c. light olive oil

Method:

1. Ahead of time, take out the egg and mustard to become room temperature.
2. Mix the mustard and egg. Slowly, pour the oil until the mixture thickens.
3. Pour in the lemon juice/vinegar. Stir well. Add a pinch of salt and pepper for additional flavoring.

Caprese Salad

Serves: 4

Nutritional Values Per Serving:

Calories: 190.75 | 63.49 g Fat | Carbohydrates: 4.58 g | Protein: 7.71 g

Ingredients:

- 3 c. grape tomatoes
- 4 peeled garlic cloves
- 2 tbsp. avocado oil
- 10 pearl-sized mozzarella balls
- 4 c. baby spinach leaves
- ¼ c. fresh basil leaves
- 1 tbsp. of each:
- -Brine reserved from the cheese
- -Pesto

Method:

1. Use aluminum foil to cover a baking tray. Program the oven to 400°F. Arrange the cloves and tomatoes on the baking pan and drizzle with the oil.
2. Bake 20-30 minutes until the tops are slightly browned.

3. Drain the liquid (saving one tablespoon) from the mozzarella. Mix the pesto with the brine.
4. Arrange the spinach in a large serving bowl. Transfer the tomatoes to the dish along with the roasted garlic. Drizzle with the pesto sauce.
5. Garnish with the mozzarella balls, and freshly torn basil leaves.

Egg Salad Stuffed Avocado

Serves: 6

Nutritional Values Per Serving:

Calories: 280.57 | Fat: 24.83 g| Carbohydrates: 3.03 g| Protein: 8.32 g

Ingredients:

- 6 large hard-boiled eggs
- 3 celery ribs
- 1/3 med. red onion
- 4 tbsp. mayonnaise
- 2 tbsp. fresh lime juice
- 2 t. brown mustard
- Pepper & salt to taste

- ½ t. cumin
- 1 t. hot sauce
- 3 med. avocados

Method:

1. Begin by chopping the onions, celery, and eggs. Discard the pit and slice the avocado in half.
2. Combine with all of the other fixings except for the avocado.
3. Scoop the salad into the avocado and serve!

Thai Pork Salad

Serves: 2

Nutritional Values Per Serving:

Calories: 461 | Fat: 32.6 g| Carbohydrates: 5.2 g| Protein: 29.2 g

Ingredients for the Salad:

- 2 c. romaine lettuce
- 10 oz. pulled pork
- ¼ medium chopped red bell pepper
- ¼ c. chopped cilantro

Ingredients for the Sauce:

- 2 tbsp. of each:
- -Tomato paste
- -Chopped cilantro
- Juice & zest of 1 lime
- 2 tbsp. (+) 2 t. soy sauce
- 1 t. of each:
- -Red curry paste
- -Five Spice
- -Fish sauce
- ¼ t. red pepper flakes
- 1 tbsp. (+) 1 t. rice wine vinegar
- ½ t. mango extract
- 10 drops liquid stevia

Method:

1. Zest half of the lime and chop the cilantro.
2. Mix all of the sauce fixings.
3. Blend the barbecue sauce components and set aside.
4. Pull the pork apart and make the salad. Pour a glaze over the pork with a bit of the sauce.

Vegetarian Club Salad

Serves: 3

Nutritional Values Per Serving:

Calories: 329.67| Fat: 26.32 g| Carbohydrates: 4.83 g| Protein: 16.82 g

Ingredients:

- 2 tbsp. of each:
- -Mayonnaise
- -Sour cream
- ½ t. of each:
- -Onion powder
- -Garlic powder
- 1 tbsp. milk
- 1 t. dried parsley
- 3 large hard-boiled eggs
- 4 oz. cheddar cheese
- ½ c. cherry tomatoes
- 1 c diced cucumber
- 3 c. torn romaine lettuce
- 1 tbsp. Dijon mustard

Method:

1. Slice the hard-boiled eggs and cube the cheese. Cut the tomatoes into halves and dice the cucumber.
2. Prepare the dressing (dried herbs, mayo, and sour cream) mixing well.
3. Add one tablespoon of milk to the mixture - and another if it's too thick.
4. Layer the salad with the vegetables, cheese, and egg slices. Scoop a spoonful of mustard in the center along with a drizzle of dressing.
5. Toss and enjoy!

Pasta

Cauliflower 'Mac N Cheese'

Serves: 4

Nutritional Values Per Serving:

Calories: 294 | Fat: 23 g| Carbohydrates: 7 g| Protein: 11 g

Ingredients:

- 3 tbsp. butter

- 1 head cauliflower
- 1 c. cheddar cheese
- Black pepper & sea salt to taste
- ¼ c. of each:
- Unsweetened almond milk
- Heavy cream

Method:

1. Cut the cauliflower into small florets and shred the cheese.
2. Prepare the oven to 450°F. Cover a baking sheet with aluminum foil or parchment paper.
3. Melt 2 tbsp. of butter. Toss the florets and butter. Give it a shake of pepper and salt. Place the cauliflower on the baking pan and roast 10-15 minutes.
4. Warm up the rest of the butter, milk, heavy cream, and cheese in the microwave or double boiler. Pour on the cheese and serve.

Fettuccine Chicken Alfredo

Serves: 2

Nutritional Values Per Serving:

Calories: 585 | Fat: 51 g| Carbohydrates: 1 g| Protein: 25 g

Ingredients:

- 2 tbsp. Macadamia nut oil
- 2 minced garlic cloves
- ½ t. dried basil
- ½ c. heavy cream
- 4 tbsp. grated parmesan

Ingredients for the Chicken and Noodles:

- 2 chicken thighs - no bones or skin
- 1 tbsp. olive oil
- 1 bag Miracle Noodle - Fettuccini
- Salt and pepper

Method:

1. ***For the Sauce***: Add the cloves to a pan with the butter for two minutes. Empty the cream into the skillet and let it simmer two additional minutes. Toss in one tablespoon of the parmesan at a time. Add the pepper, salt, and dried

basil. Simmer three to five minutes on the low heat setting.
2. ***For the Chicken:*** Pound the chicken with a meat tenderizer hammer until it is approximately ½-inch thick. Warm up the oil in a skillet using the medium heat setting and put the chicken in to cook for about seven minutes per side. Shred and set aside.
3. ***For the Noodles:*** Prepare the package of noodles. Rinse, and boil them for two minutes in a pot of water.
4. Fold in the noodles along with the sauce and shredded chicken. Cook slowly for two minutes and enjoy.

Lemon Garlic Shrimp Pasta

Serves: 4
Nutritional Values Per Serving:
Calories: 360| Fat: 21 g| Carbohydrates: 3.5 g| Protein: 36 g

Ingredients:

- 2 bags angel hair pasta
- 4 garlic cloves
- 2 tbsp. each:
- Olive oil
- Macadamia oil
- ½ lemon
- 1 lb. large raw shrimp
- ½ t. paprika
- Fresh basil
- Pepper and salt

Method:

1. Drain the water from the package of noodles and rinse them in cold water. Add them to a pot of boiling water for two minutes. Transfer them to a hot skillet over medium heat to remove the excess liquid (dry roast). Set them to the side.
2. Use the same pan to warm the oil, and smashed garlic. Saute a few minutes but don't brown.
3. Slice the lemon into rounds and add them to the garlic along with the shrimp. Saute for approximately three minutes per side.
4. Add the noodles and spices and stir to blend the flavors.

Pizza

BBQ Meat-Lover's Pizza

Serves: 2

Nutritional Values Per Serving:

Calories: 205| Fat: 27 g| Carbohydrates: 3.5 g| Protein: 18 g

Ingredients:

- 2 c. (8 oz.) mozzarella
- 1 tbsp. psyllium husk powder
- ¾ c. almond flour
- 3 tbsp. (1 ½ oz.) cream cheese
- 1 large egg
- ½ t. of each:
- Black pepper
- Salt
- 1 tbsp. Italian seasoning

Ingredients for the Topping:

- 1 c. (4 oz.) mozzarella cheese
- To Taste: BBQ sauce
- Sliced Kabana/hard salami
- Bacon slices
- Sprinkled oregano - optional

Method:

1. Set the temperature of the oven to 400°F.
2. Melt the cheese in the microwave until it melts – about 45 seconds. Toss in the cream cheese and egg, mixing well.
3. Blend in the psyllium husk, flour, salt, pepper, and Italian seasoning. Make the dough as circular as possible. Bake for ten minutes. Flip it onto a piece of parchment paper.
4. Cover the crust with the toppings and some more cheese. Bake until the cheese is golden, slice, and serve.

Beef Pizza

Serves: 4

Nutritional Values Per Serving:

Calories: 610| Fat: 45 g |Carbohydrates: 2 g | Protein: 44 g

Ingredients:

- 2 large eggs
- 1 pkg. (20 oz.) ground beef
- 28 pepperoni slices
- ½ c. of each:
- Shredded cheddar cheese
- Pizza sauce
- 4 oz. mozzarella cheese
- Also Needed: 1 Cast iron skillet

Method:

1. Combine the eggs, beef, and seasonings. Place in the skillet to form the crust. Bake until the meat is done or about 15 minutes.
2. Take it out and add the sauce, cheese, and toppings. Place the pizza in the oven a few minutes until the cheese has melted. Remove and enjoy!

Bell Pepper Basil Pizza

Servings: 4 - 2 Pizzas

Nutritional values per serving:

Calories: 411.5| Fat: 31.32 g| Carbohydrates: 6.46 g| Protein: 22.26 g

Ingredients for the Pizza Base:

- 6 oz. mozzarella cheese
- 2 tbsp. of each:
- -Fresh parmesan cheese
- -Cream cheese
- Psyllium Husk
- 1 t. Italian seasoning
- 1 large egg
- ½ t. of each:
- Black pepper
- Salt

Ingredients for the Toppings:

- 4 oz. shredded cheddar cheese
- ¼ c. marinara sauce
- 1 med. vine ripened tomato
- 2-3 med. bell peppers
- 2-3 tbsp. fresh basil – chopped

Method:

1. Set the temperature in the oven to 400°F.
2. Melt the cheese in the microwave until melted and pliable or for 40-50 seconds. Add the remainder of the pizza base fixings to the cheese – mixing well with your hands.
3. Flatten the dough to form the two circular pizzas. Bake ten minutes. Remove and add the toppings. Take for about 8-10 additional minutes.
4. Let it cool and serve.

Pita Pizza

Serves: 2

Nutritional Values Per Serving:

Calories: 250| Fat: 19 g| Carbohydrates: 4 g| Protein: 13 g

Ingredients:

- ½ c. marinara sauce
- 1 low-carb pita
- 2 oz. cheddar cheese
- 14 slices pepperoni
- 1 oz. roasted red peppers

Method:

1. Set the oven to 450°F.
2. Slice the pita in half and put on a foil-lined baking tray. Rub with a bit of oil and toast for one to two minutes.
3. Pour the sauce over the bread, sprinkle with the cheese, and other toppings. Bake for another five minutes or until the cheese melts.

Tacos & Wraps

Chipotle Fish Tacos

Serves: 4
Nutritional values per serving:
Calories: 300 | Fat: 20 g| Carbohydrates: 7 g| Protein: 24 g

Ingredients:

- ½ small diced yellow onion
- 2 pressed cloves of garlic
- 1 chopped fresh jalapeno
- 2 tbsp. olive oil
- 4 oz. chipotle peppers in adobo sauce
- 2 tbsp. each:
- -Mayonnaise
- -macadamia nut oil
- 4 low-carb tortillas
- 1 lb. haddock fillet's

Method:
1. In a skillet, fry the onion on med-high for five minutes.
2. Lower the temperature to the medium heat setting. Toss in the garlic, and jalapeno. Stir another two minutes.
3. Chop and add the chipotles, along with the adobo sauce into the pan.
4. Drop the butter, mayonnaise, and fish into the pan and cook about eight minutes.
5. Make the Tacos: Fry the tortilla for approximately two minutes for each side. Chill and shape them with the prepared fixings.

Cumin Spiced Beef Wraps

Serves: 2

Nutritional Values Per Serving:

Calories: 375| Fat: 26 g| Carbohydrates: 4 g| Protein: 30 g

Ingredients:

- 1-2 tbsp. coconut oil
- ¼ onion – diced
- 2/3 lb. ground beef
- 2 tbsp. chopped cilantro
- 1 diced red bell pepper
- 1 t. minced ginger
- 2 t. cumin
- 4 minced garlic cloves
- Pepper and salt to your liking
- 8 large cabbage leaves

Method:

1. Warm up a frying pan and pour in the oil. Sauté the peppers, onions, and ground beef using medium heat.

When done, add the pepper, salt, cumin, ginger, cilantro, and garlic.

2. Fill a large pot with water (3/4 full) and wait for it to boil. Cook each leaf for 20 seconds, plunge it in cold water and drain before placing it on your serving dish.
3. Scoop the mixture onto each leaf, fold, and enjoy.

Dinner

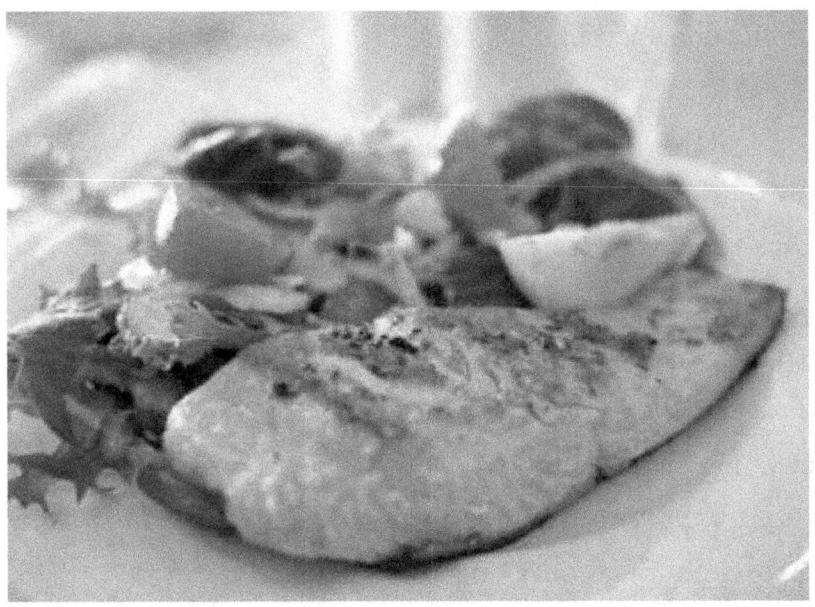

Beef for Dinner

Balsamic Beef Pot Roast

Serves: 10

Nutritional Values Per Serving:

Calories: 393 | Fat: 28g| Carbohydrates: 3 g| Protein: 30 g

Ingredients:

- 1 boneless (approx. 3 lb.) chuck roast
- 1 t. of each:
- -Garlic powder
- -Black ground pepper
- 1 tbsp. kosher salt
- ¼ c. balsamic vinegar
- ½ c. chopped onion
- 2 c. water
- ¼ t. xanthan gum

For the Garnish:

- Freshly chopped parsley

Method:

1. Combine the salt, garlic powder, and pepper and rub the chuck roast with the combined fixings.
2. Use a heavy skillet to sear the roast. Add the vinegar and deglaze the pan as you continue cooking for one more minute.
3. Toss the onion into a pot with the (two cups) boiling water along with the roast. Cover with a top and simmer for three to four hours on a low setting.
4. Take the meat from the pot and add to a cutting surface. Shred into chunks and remove any fat or bones.
5. Add the xanthan gum to the broth and whisk. Place the roast meat back in the pan to warm up.
6. Serve with a favorite side dish.

Cheeseburger Calzone

Serves: 8
Nutritional Values Per Serving:
Calories: 580| Fat: 47 g| Carbohydrates: 3 g| Protein: 34 g

Ingredients:

- ½ yellow diced onion
- 1 ½ lb. ground beef – lean
- 4 thick-cut bacon strips
- 4 dill pickle spears
- 8 oz. cream cheese – divided
- 1 egg
- ½ c. mayonnaise
- 1 c. of each:
- -Shredded cheddar cheese
- -Almond flour
- -Shredded mozzarella cheese

Method:

1. Program the oven to 425°F. Prepare a cookie tin with parchment paper.
2. Chop the pickles into spears. Set aside for now.
3. Prepare the Crust: Combine ½ of the cream cheese and the mozzarella cheese. Microwave 35 seconds. When it melts, add the egg and almond flour to make the dough. Set aside.
4. Cook the beef on the stove using medium heat.
5. Cook the bacon (microwave for five minutes or stovetop). When cool, break into bits.

6. Dice the onion and add to the beef and cook until softened. Toss in the bacon, cheddar cheese, pickle bits, the rest of the cream cheese, and mayonnaise. Stir well.
7. Roll the dough onto the prepared baking tin. Scoop the mixture into the center. Fold the ends and side to make the calzone.
8. Bake until browned or about 15 minutes. Let it rest for 10 minutes before slicing.

Nacho Steak in the Skillet

Serves: 5
Nutritional Values Per Serving:
Calories: 385.4| Fat: 30.67 g| Carbohydrates: 5.9 g| Protein: 18.87 g

Ingredients:

- 1 tbsp. butter
- 8 oz. beef round tip steak
- 1/3 c. melted refined coconut oil
- ½ t. turmeric
- 1 t. chili powder
- 1 ½ pounds cauliflower
- 1 oz. each shredded:
- -Cheddar cheese
- -Monterey Jack cheese

Possible Garnishes:

- 1 oz. canned jalapeno slices
- 1/3 c. sour cream
- Avocado – Approx. 5 oz.

Method:

1. Set the oven temperature to 400°F.
2. Prepare the cauliflower into chip-like shapes.
3. Combine the turmeric, chili powder, and coconut oil in a mixing dish.
4. Toss in the cauliflower and add it to a tin. Set the baking timer for 20 to 25 minutes.
5. Over med-high heat in a cast iron skillet, add the butter. Cook until both sides are done, flipping just once. Let it rest for five to ten minutes. Thinly slice, and sprinkle with some pepper and salt to the steak.
6. When done, transfer the florets to the skillet and add the steak strips. Top it off with the cheese and bake five to ten more minutes.
7. Serve with your favorite garnish but count those carbs.

Portobello Bun Cheeseburgers

Serves: 6

Nutritional Values Per Serving:

Calories: 336| Fat: 22.8 g| Carbohydrates: 4 g| Protein: 29.1 g

Ingredients:

- 1 lb. ground beef - lean 80/20
- 1 t. of each:
- 1 tbsp. Worcestershire sauce
- -Pink Himalayan salt
- -Ground black pepper
- 1 tbsp. avocado oil
- 6 slices sharp cheddar cheese
- 6 Portobello mushroom caps

Method:

1. Remove the stem, rinse, and dab dry the mushrooms.
2. Combine the salt, pepper, beef, and Worcestershire sauce in a mixing container. Form into patties.
3. Warm up the oil (medium heat). Let the caps simmer about three to four minutes per side.

4. Transfer the mushrooms to a bowl - using the same pan - cook the patties four minutes, flip, and cook another five minutes until done.
5. Add the cheese to the burgers and cover for one minute to melt the cheese.
6. Add one of the mushroom caps to the burgers along with the desired garnishes and serve.

Steak-Lovers Slow-Cooked Chili in the Slow Cooker

Serves: 12

Nutritional Values Per Serving:

Calories: 321| Fat: 26 g| Carbohydrates: 3.3 g| Protein: 38.4 g

With Toppings:

Calories: 540.3| Fat: 41.32 g| Carbohydrates: 13.49 g| Protein: 32.47 g

Ingredients for the Chili:

- 1 c. beef or chicken stock
- ½ c. sliced leeks
- 2 ½ lbs. (1-inch cubes) steak
- 2 c. whole tomatoes (canned with juices)

- 1/8 t. black pepper
- ½ t. salt
- ½ t. cumin
- ¼ t. ground cayenne pepper
- 1 tbsp. chili powder

Optional Toppings:

- 1 t. fresh chopped cilantro
- 2 tbsp. sour cream
- ¼ c/ shredded cheddar cheese
- ½ avocado – sliced or cubed

Method:

1. Toss all of the fixings into the cooker - except the toppings.
2. Use the cooker's high setting for about six hours.
3. Serve, add the toppings, and enjoy.

Vegetarian Keto Burger on a Bun

Serves: 2

Nutritional Values Per Serving:

Calories: 637| Fat: 55.1 g| Carbohydrates: 8.7 g| Protein: 23.7 g

Mushroom Ingredients:

- 1-2 tbsp. freshly chopped basil – 1 t. dried
- 2 medium-large flat mushrooms – ex. Portobello
- 1 tbsp. of each:
- -Coconut oil/ghee
- -Freshly chopped oregano – ½ t. dried
- 1 crushed garlic clove
- ¼ t. salt
- Black pepper

Serving Ingredients:

- 2 large organic eggs
- 2 slices cheddar/gouda cheese
- 2 tbsp. mayonnaise
- 2 keto buns – see recipe below

Also Needed:

1 griddle pan/regular skillet

Method:

1. Prepare the mushrooms for marinating by seasoning with crushed garlic, pepper, salt, ghee (melted), and fresh herbs. Save a small amount for frying the eggs. Marinate for about one hour at room temperature.
2. Arrange the mushrooms in the pan with the top side facing upwards. Cook for about five minutes on the med-high setting. Flip and continue cooking for another five minutes.
3. Remove the pan from the burner and flip the mushrooms over and add the cheese. When it is time to serve, put them under the broiler for a minute or so to melt the cheese.
4. With the remainder of the ghee, fry the eggs leaving the yolk runny. Remove from the heat.
5. Slice the buns and add them to the grill, cooking until crisp for about two to three minutes.
6. To assemble, add one tablespoon of mayonnaise to each bun and top them off with the mushroom, egg, tomato, and lettuce.
7. Put the tops on the buns (see recipe below) and serve.

Keto Buns for the Burger

Serves: 12

Nutritional Values Per Serving:

Calories: 189| Fat: 12.6 g| Carbohydrates: 3.1 g| Protein: 11.6 g

Note: Erythritol has 0.4 g carbohydrates, and Xylitol has 10 g.

Dry Ingredients:

- ½ c. of each:
- -Ground sesame/poppy seeds
- -Flax meal
- -Unflavored whey protein/egg white protein powder
- 1 c. of each:
- -Almond flour
- -Coconut flour
- 1 tbsp. of each:
- -Dried oregano
- -Minced garlic
- -Cream of tartar
- -Xylitol or Erythritol
- 2 tsp. baking soda
- 1 tsp. salt

Wet Ingredients:

- 2 large eggs
- 6 large egg whites
- 1 tbsp. extra-virgin coconut oil
- 2 c. hot water

Method:

1. Prepare the oven temperature to 350°F.
2. Toss the sesame seeds in a processor and pulse until powdery. Blend in all of the dry components, omitting the coconut flour for now. Mix well.
3. Combine the hot water and eggs. Add to the dry fixings, mixing well. Gradually combine the coconut flour until you have a dense uniformity. Be sure not to make the mixture too dry.
4. Scoop the dough onto a baking pan - leaving them several inches apart and sprinkle with the poppy/sesame seeds. Bake for 20-30 minutes or until browned.

Chicken for Dinner

Barbecue Pulled Chicken in the Slow Cooker

Serves: 8

Nutritional Values Per Serving:

Calories: 219| Fat: 7.2 g| Carbohydrates: 4.3 g| Protein: 33.8 g

Ingredients:

- 3 lb. chicken thighs
- 1 t. of each:
- -Cumin
- -Smoked paprika
- -Onion powder
- ¼ t. pepper
- ¾ t. salt - divided
- 1 t. maple extract
- ¼ c. apple cider vinegar
- 1 c. sugar-free ketchup
- ½ c. water
- ½ t. clear liquid stevia
- 1 tbsp. unsweetened cocoa powder
- ¼ t. cumin

Method:

1. Remove all of the bones and chicken and arrange the chicken on a baking sheet. Combine the salt, pepper, cumin, onion powder, and paprika together. Rub it over the chicken.
2. Pour the ketchup, vinegar, and water into the slow cooker. Stir, and add the rest of the fixings. Lastly, add the chicken.
3. Close the lid and cook four hours on high or eight hours on low.
4. Enjoy over some rice (add the carbs).

Chicken Parmesan

Serves: 2

Nutritional Values Per Serving:

Calories: 600| Fat: 32 g| Carbohydrates: 3 g| Protein: 74 g

Ingredients:

- 1 lb. breasts of chicken
- 2 tbsp. parmesan cheese
- 1 oz. pork rinds
- 1 egg

- ½ c. of each:
- -Marinara sauce
- -Shredded mozzarella

Possible Garnish Ingredients:

- -Pepper and salt
- -Garlic powder
- -Oregano

Method:

1. Program the oven temperature to 350°F.
2. Use a food processor/Magic Bullet to crush the pork rinds and parmesan cheese. Add them to a bowl.
3. Pound the chicken breasts until they are ½-inch thick. Beat the egg and dip the chicken in for an egg wash. Dip the chicken into the crumbs.
4. Arrange the breasts on a lightly greased baking sheet. Sprinkle with the seasonings and bake 25 minutes.
5. Dump the marinara sauce over each portion. Garnish with the mozzarella and bake for 15 minutes.
6. Enjoy with a bed of spinach.

Coconut Curry Chicken Tenders

Serves: 5
Nutritional Values Per Serving:
Calories: 494 | Fat: 39.4 g| Carbohydrates: 2.1 g| Protein: 29.4 g

Ingredients for the Tenders:

- 1 large egg
- 1 pkg. chicken thighs (24 oz.) deboned with skin /5 thighs
- ½ c. of each:
- -Crumbled pork rinds (1 ½ oz.)
- -Unsweetened shredded coconut
- 1/2 t. coriander
- 2 t. curry powder
- ¼ t. of each:
- -Onion powder
- -Garlic powder
- Pepper & salt to your liking

Sweet and Spicy Mango Dipping Sauce Ingredients:

- ¼ c. of each:
- -Sour cream
- -Mayonnaise
- 1 ½ t. mango extract
- 2 tbsp. sugar-free ketchup
- ¼ t. cayenne pepper
- ½ t. of each:
- -Ground ginger
- -Garlic powder
- -Red pepper flakes
- 7 drops liquid stevia

Method:

1. Set the oven to 400°F.
2. Whisk the eggs and debone the thighs. Slice them into strips (skins on).
3. Add the spices, coconut, and pork rinds to a Ziploc-type bag. Add the chicken, shake, and place on a wire rack. Bake for about 15 minutes. Flip them over and continue baking for another 20 minutes.
4. Combine the sauce components and stir well. Serve with your piping hot chicken tenders

Pizza Chicken Casserole in the Slow Cooker

Serves: 3

Nutritional Values Per Serving:

Calories: 228 | Fat: 8.8 g| Carbohydrates: 6 g| Protein: 31.2 g

Ingredients:

- 2 cubed chicken breasts
- 1 can tomato sauce – 8 oz.
- 1 t. Italian seasoning
- 1 bay leaf
- Dash of pepper
- ¼ t. salt
- To Garnish: ½ c. shredded mozzarella cheese
- Recommended: 2-quart slow cooker

Method:

1. Remove the bones from the chicken and chop into cubes. Add them to the slow cooker.
2. Pour in the sauce over the chicken and add the spices. Stir and cook on the low setting for three to four hours.
3. Serve with the cheese as a garnish.

Conclusion

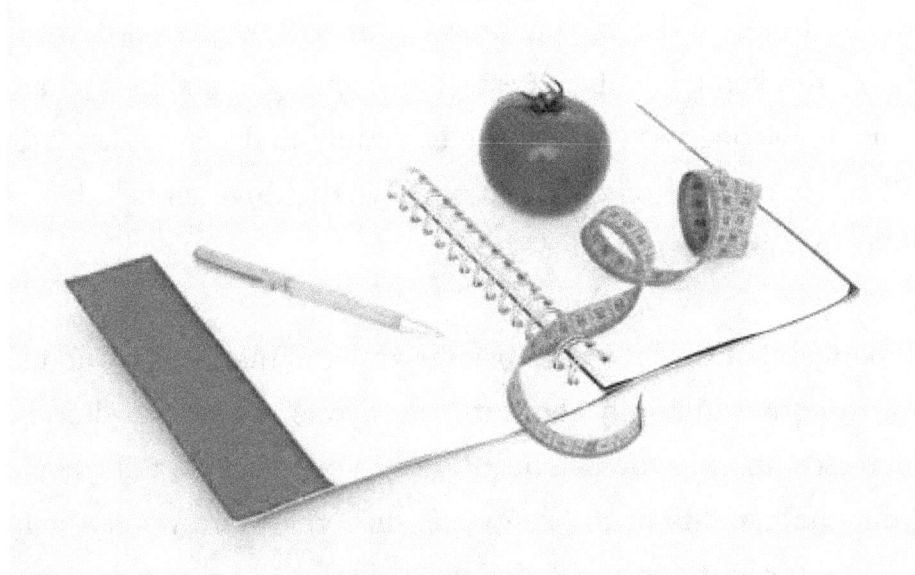

Thank you so much for making it all the way to the end of this book. We hope that you have found a treasure trove of information which is certain to help you keep those unwanted pounds off. Best of all, you don't need any special science or equipment. You have everything you need in order to make the best of your personal abilities to follow this eating plan.

Indeed, the road to health and wellbeing has its ups and downs; in fact, we all go through them. There is no arguing that. But what truly counts is your motivation and desire to stay on track despite any drawbacks. We sincerely hope that attitude has come across throughout this book.

Please go over this book as repetition is the best way in which we are able to learn. Before you know it, you will be an expert in the arts of the ketogenic diet. Best of all, you will be able to share your knowledge with your friends, family and colleagues. You will surely be able to help them improve their overall health and wellbeing just like you have.

If you feel that this book has been useful and informative, do tell your friends and family about it… or anyone you think would be interested in this topic. The more we are able to tell people about the benefits of the ketogenic diet, the more we can help others improve their health and wellbeing.

What could be better than that?

Thanks again. Hope to see you in the next one.

INTERMITTENT FASTING OVER 50

The Ultimate and Complete Guide for Healthy Weight Loss, Burn Fat, Slow Aging, Detox Your Body and Support Your Hormones with the Process of Metabolic Autophagy

INTRODUCTION

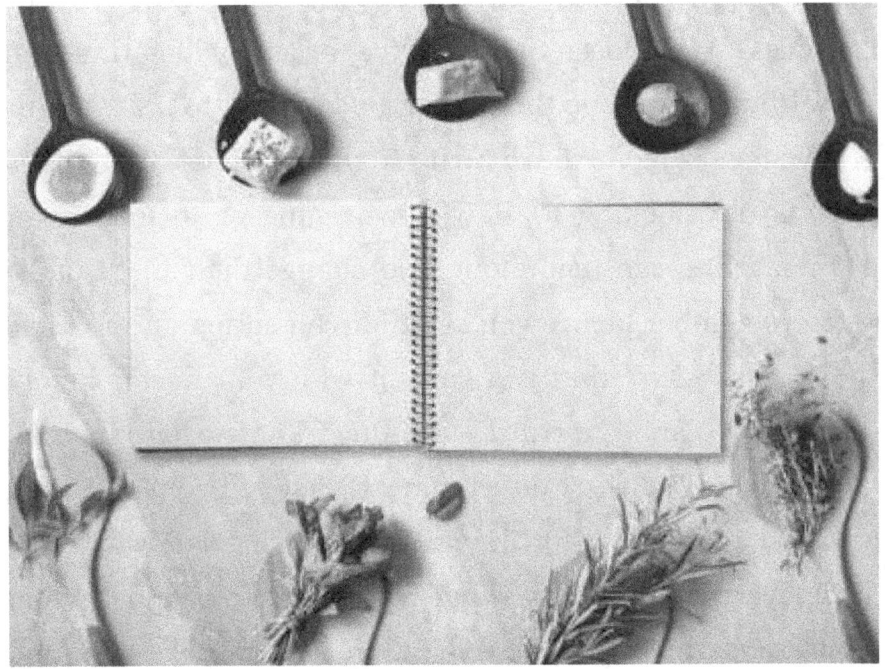

Thank you so much for purchasing the *Intermittent Fasting Over 50: The Ultimate and Complete Guide for Healthy Weight Loss, Burn Fat, Slow Aging, Detox Your Body, and Support Your Hormones with the Process of Metabolic Autophagy.* In this book, we will talk about intermittent fasting, more specifically on how someone should follow intermittent fasting if they are above the age of 50.

Many people don't realize it, but intermittent fasting is fantastic for people who are above the age of 50 as it helps them to slow down aging and detoxify their bodies. One of the main things to worry about once you get up to the age of 50 is that you need healing the body the right way so that you can slow down the aging process. Who doesn't want to live for a very long time and to be healthy at the same time. Everybody wants to achieve this goal, which is why we have written this book so that many people who are looking to slow down aging or to feel better about themselves can read along and change their life. Couple things to remember before you start implementing and reading this book, make sure that you consult with your doctor before you begin any plan. The truth is we don't know what situation you are in, which is why we recommend that you consult with a professional before you start intermittent fasting as it cannot be ideal for everyone. Another thing to remember would be that intermittent fasting has to be done correctly, so make sure that you understand everything in this book before you start implementing the tips and tricks. Other than that, you should be good to go when it comes to intermittent fasting.

Chapter 1: What Is Intermittent Fasting?

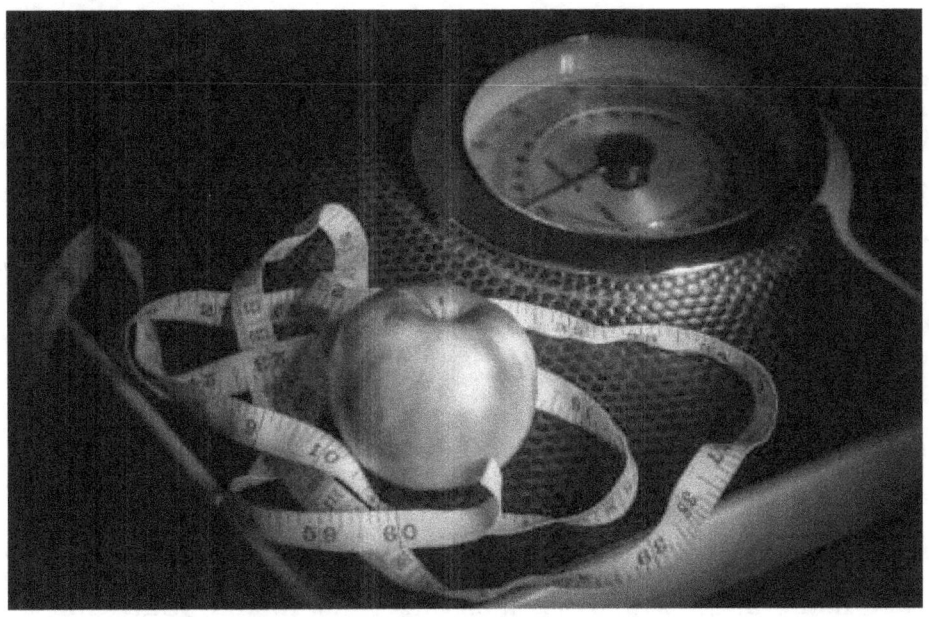

In this chapter, we will talk about intermittent fasting and what it means to follow intermittent fasting. If you have been living under a rock, there's a high chance that you have no idea what intermittent fasting is or what it can do for you. What we will do is go through the basics of intermittent fasting so that you understand what intermittent fasting is and that you have a better understanding of it moving on. A quick disclaimer, this chapter might be boring too many people as the information is very remedial. However, this information to some might be new, so if you find this chapter boring, then you are free to skip it. However, if you're still iffy about intermittent fasting or that you have no idea on exactly what it does, then we recommend that you stick around. Time and time again, people have followed different types of fad diets, which may or may not work for them. Even if they do work for them, chances are they would give up very quickly and gain back the weight or the results that they achieved. The reason why they would give up and go back to the normal cell is that it is straightforward not to make it a habit or to make it a lifestyle.

The problem with modern-day and fad diets is that it is simply not sustainable in the long-term. If you want to lose weight and feel better by yourself for the rest of your life, then you need to pick something which is not only sustainable but can be adjusted into your lifestyle based on your needs. Moreover, you need something that gives you the freedom to eat and have whatever it is that you like in moderation so that you can enjoy life and be with your friends and family a lot more often. The truth is, many fad diets do not allow you to eat food, which is unhealthy. Don't get me wrong; eating unhealthy food all the time is not the best thing for your body anyways.

However, we recommend that you eat decent quality food often so that you see the benefits that you are looking for when it comes to losing fat or building muscle. However, eating decent food all the time can be a tedious task, which can lead to failure in the long-term, which is why having unhealthy food which tastes good here and there can lead to overall success in the long-term. With that being said, following fat diets play does not allow you to eat anything which is unhealthy. Most of the time, the fad diets put you in a position where you are insanely starving your body. Starving your body in the short-term might lead to weight loss, which might make you feel better, however starving yourself in the long-term can lead to many unwanted health fallbacks.

This is another reason why people who start following fad diets tend to give up so soon. This is where intermittent fasting comes in; the great thing about intermittent fasting is that many people don't even switch up what they are eating. What they do is eat cyclically. They would eat for certain hours of the day and would not eat for certain hours of the day. In essence, intermittent fasting is a cyclical way of eating. Now the most common way for people to follow intermittent fasting would be the 16/8 method. And this method you will be eating for 8 hours of the day, and you will be fasting for 16 hours of the day.

This is where you will not get any food to eat, and we'll have to survive on water or black coffee. You can have anything you want, which has no calories when you are fasting. Now there are tons of intermittent fasting methods which we will talk about later on in this book. However, the 16/8 method has been working very well for most people and can be added to their lifestyle. The great thing about this method would be that you don't have to worry about having certain hours to be more important than others when it comes to eating window and visa-versa. You will be the one picking out the times for your eating window and your fasting window. The most common times for fasting are 8 pm till 12 pm the next day, then eating from 12 pm to 8 pm, again this time could be whatever works for your schedule.

Another great thing about intermittent fasting would be that there are no restrictions on what you could be eating. For example, during the eating window, many people eat whatever they want within reason to achieve their goals. I have seen many Fitness professionals eat food such as buttermilk biscuit, or even candy and dessert sometimes during the eating window, and still lose weight. We don't recommend you do that. However, this plan gives you the freedom to eat whatever you want while still seeing the results when it comes to losing fat and building muscle.

If you want to lose fat even more efficiently when intermittent fasting, we recommend that you eat a good, well-balanced diet slightly in a caloric deficit. This will allow you to not only lose fat but also to be certain that you're going to see results in the long-term when it comes to overall health and well-being. We also recommend that you accompany this with a fitness plan, make sure that you're working out in the gym if you want to lose fat and see the results that you have been hoping for. Another great thing about intermittent fasting, especially for people who are over the age of 50 years, is that it slows aging. One of the very best things, when it comes to intermittent fasting would be that it allows you to have very well-balanced aging and to make you look younger. These are thanks to two things, and the first one would be the increase in growth hormone. As you may know, intermittent fasting has shown to increase growth hormone production. This hormone is the youth of foundation, the reason why is because it will help you to recover quickly.

The benefits of growth hormone also include better skin and better bones, and you will also lose more fat and build more muscle. Another thing that intermittent fasting helps with would be the process known as autophagy. Autophagy is a process where your body gets rid of old/dead cells and replaces them with new cells.

This is the reason why you see the youth benefits, and also the reason why many people stay young for a very long time. These detoxifying cells would also mean getting rid of any diseased cells, which may include cancerous cells. Many people claim to get rid of their cancer very quickly by following intermittent fasting, and we can't back that up; however, it has been claimed by many cancer survivors. If you're someone looking to not only be better when it comes to Performance inside and outside the gym but also to look a lot younger in the long-term, then you have no reason why not to follow intermittent fasting. We will make it very easy for you when it comes to picking out the right plan and how to follow it appropriately.

Understand this, and intermittent fasting could be one of the easiest plans you could follow. And it all starts by reading this book. Do you have already taken the first step to seeing better results with your body and health, so make sure that you go all the way with it. Intermittent fasting is like eating in increments. As we told you, it is a cyclical way of eating food, which allows you to consume all the calories you need in a certain hour of the day. While certain of the day, you will be fasting and not eating anything at all. Once you start following intermittent fasting, you will be surprised how much time we spend on eating food. We spend a lot of time, more specifically waste a lot of time eating food. If you're someone who is looking to see success with their business or their work environment, then you will gain from that time and see the results that you have been hoping for. Intermittent fasting truly is a win-win situation. It makes you feel younger, and it gets rid of any bad cells in your body while increasing all the good hormones. Think of it this way, and there are many people who follow intermittent fasting without even knowing it. Many religions recommend that you fast for 30 days, or however long. This goes to show intermittent fasting has been in practice for a very long time, and good reason, it simply works.

Now, if you are someone who can't fast every day for the rest of your life, don't worry as you will have at least one day in the week or you can eat throughout the whole day. We recommend that you do that as it will allow you to be more motivated in the long-term, which is what intermittent fasting is all about is creating a lifestyle. If you are tired of following diets that yield you some results, but they aren't sustainable in the long-term, then chances are intermittent fasting is going to be your savior.

Make sure that you pick the plan that fits your needs and your goals. We will talk about all the intermittent fasting methods later on in this book. However, once you understand the benefits and the reasons why you need to be following intermittent fasting, then it will be straightforward for you to follow it in the long-term. The main thing that differentiates intermittent fasting to any other fad diet is that they're health benefits to intermittent fasting and not just aesthetic benefits. Meaning, God guides give you a set of promises which may or may not be delivered. However, intermittent fasting has shown time and time again to deliver aesthetic benefits, and on top of that, help you get rid of many diseases that will help you stay healthy for a very long time.

Intermittent fasting is also one of the best plans to follow up for someone who's over the age of 50. The reasons why we told you is because it helps you to say younger and to enjoy life a lot more when you're 50 the main thing you want to do is enjoy the life, if you want to enjoy life then you need to be in a healthy State of Mind and Body. Intermittent fasting gives you all of that, and on top of that, it helps you to say a lot younger for a very long time. If you don't believe me, then look at your celebrities, many celebrities who are in their 50s tend to follow intermittent fasting and for an excellent reason. It is because it helps them to stay younger and to think a lot better and quickly.

Finally, intermittent fasting helps you to save a lot more time because you will not be thinking about eating for a certain amount of time, which will allow you to spend that time working on your craft. With that being said, we now conclude this chapter. The main take-home message from this chapter would be that intermittent fasting can be used for numerous reasons, if you are someone looking to gain muscle or lose fat or you want to be younger for a long time. Also, intermittent fasting is something that should be considered more of a lifestyle than something which is to be done once every two months. Now, if you are serious about changing your life, and about starting living healthier than intermittent fasting is the answer for you.

Chapter 2: Benefits of Intermittent Fasting

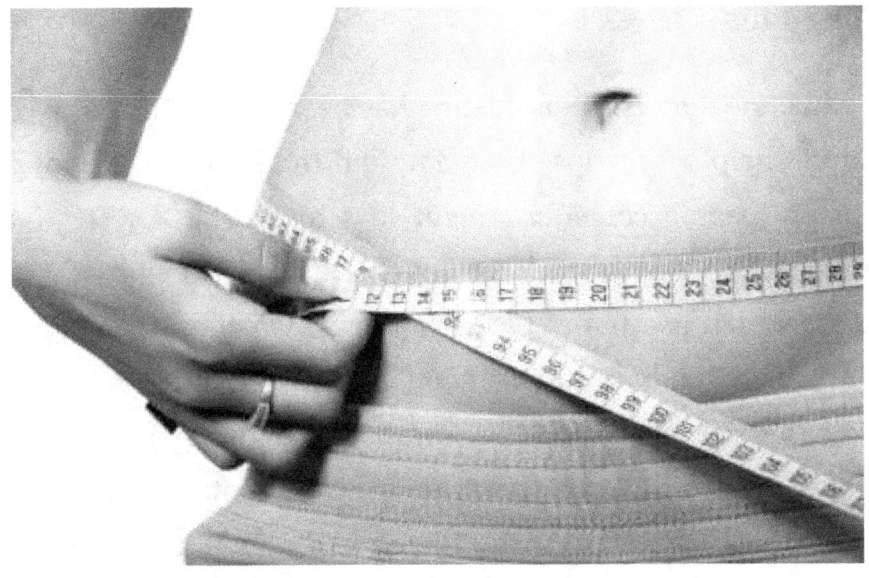

Now that you have a clear idea of what intermittent fasting is, let's talk about some of the benefits that come along with intermittent fasting. The truth is many benefits come along with intermittent fasting, and they have all of them backed up by science. Keeping that in mind, we will now talk about some of the significant benefits which come along with intermittent fasting so that you can get a better idea of why you should follow it and how it can be beneficial to you. One thing to remember is that all these benefits are great, but you must make sure that you are fit to follow intermittent fasting if you're not fit and healthy to support intermittent fasting than we would advise you not to follow it. The best way to find out if you can observe intermittent fasting is to consult with your doctor before you do any such plans, enough of that let's get into the topic of benefits.

Weight loss

As you know, intermittent fasting has been shown time and time again to help people lose body fat, and the keyword is body fat, as many people consider weight loss to be the key. If you're losing muscle, then there's no benefit of losing weight, as losing muscle can cause many health hazards. On the other hand, if you're losing body fat, then it could be perfect for you as it can lower the risk of many other diseases that come along. Many people who start falling intermittent fasting notice a decrease in body fat, and the reason why that is is that you are not spiking your insulin all the time and converting all those carbs into fat.

As you know, when you eat anything, your insulin goes up, and if it does not have time to use up all those calories in glycogen, it will be stored into fat. The great thing about intermittent fasting is that you don't have to worry about getting all those glycogens stored into fat as you will not be eating so frequently. When you're not eating so often, then you will start burning body fat that you already have. They're for preserving your muscles while using body fat for the energy source. The great thing about that is, you will not be using any glycogen at all and merely be burning off that excess body fat. You see, when you're intermittent fasting, your body goes into starvation mode, which is healthy for you. We have evolved to live without food for a couple of days, so it is our natural habitat not to eat food all the time. What intermittent fasting does helps us with our back in the daily routine and use body fat for energy?

Muscle gain

There have been many studies showing that intermittent fasting can help you put on muscle, and the truth is that intermittent fasting is perfect for putting on muscle and losing body fat. When you're intermittent fasting, your body will be increasing your hormone production of growth hormone and testosterone. Especially in men, which is why intermittent fasting is the ideal scenario for natural athletes to put on muscle. If you're someone who's abusing steroids, then there's no benefit for you to use intermittent fasting when it comes to putting on muscle. However, if you use the healthy route and not use any steroids, then intermittent fasting can be the answer for you. When you're intermittent fasting, your growth hormone can go up to 4000% office natural levels.

As you know, growth hormone has been shown to put on and preserve muscle while increasing your bone density. This is a no-brainer for natural athletes, as you will be increasing your testosterone and growth hormone at the same time you will put on muscle. On the other hand, you will also be cleaning out your gut, which will help you digest food a lot more efficiently. Many people don't know this. Still, intermittent fasting can help you clean out your stomach, having a healthy gut is very important when you're looking towards putting on muscle so make sure that you consider that when starting any muscle gaining plan.

Mental fog.

Intermittent fasting has also been shown to reduce mental fog. As you know, mental fog can be one of the most annoying things you can face when you're trying to achieve something in your work or personal life. What intermittent fasting does is help you not worry about digesting and focus on feeding your brain. Let me explain when you're eating all the time your body concentrated on understanding the food. When you're intermittent fasting body does not have to worry about food and in fact, give you the mental focus you need. Most of the time, people cannot focus on is because they don't have the energy to concentrate as their body is digesting their food. As simple as a sound, but it's true when you're not understanding, you are a lot more focused on the work that you're doing only because your body has nothing else to do. If your organization is free of any digestion on any other thing that it has to focus on, that's when you can take up all the things you want to do, so if you're going to focus a lot more and rid of the mental fog, your body will facilitate that for you very directly. Also, there have been many scientific studies showing that intermittent fasting, along with ketogenic diet, can help you tremendously to focus. As you know, insulin production can help us feel a lot more lethargic, which is why when following a ketogenic diet and intermittent fasting, insulin levels won't be out of whack. Therefore, you will have a lot less mental fog and a lot more mental clarity and focus.

Reduce blood pressure:

As you know, intermittent fasting as shown to reduce blood pressure, which makes it an excellent plan for people to follow when it comes to putting on muscle and losing body fat. If you're eating a lot more food, which should be our goal when it comes to putting on muscle, then chances are your blood pressure will be going up. However, when you're following intermittent fasting, that's something you don't have to worry about it, like intermittent fasting, as shown to reduce blood pressure. There have been many scientific studies showing that intermittent fasting can and will lower blood pressure. So it is one of the best things to follow when it comes to lowering your blood pressure and to see better health benefits overall. Whether it is your goal to lose fat or build muscle having a lower blood pressure is very crucial for you as well help your cardiovascular health and wellness. Cardiovascular health and wellness are essential as a house you live a long, fruitful life, so keep that into consideration when following intermittent fasting.

Lower cholesterol levels

Recently there was a 3-week study showing that intermittent fasting can reduce cholesterol levels tremendously. In the study, it showed that people reduce their bad cholesterol by a couple of points. Without getting to sign to pick on you, intermittent fasting has been scientifically proven to lower the bad cholesterol in your body. If you are facing cholesterol issues, then definitely consider intermittent fasting as a can help you with lowering cholesterol levels. Cholesterol is a silent killer in the United States, which is why it is essential to understand how cholesterol works and how it can help you or hinder you. Meaning the right amount of natural cholesterol level is critical, however when it gets too high, and it is mostly the wrong cholesterol level, then the chances are that you are not in the right place when it comes to health. Which is why it is essential to understand how cholesterol levels work and how to reduce them, if you're following intermittent fasting then that's something you don't have to worry about as it does everything for you.

Cancer

Intermittent fasting is also shown to reduce the risk of cancer. As you know, cancer grows in our body very rapidly. There have been many scientific studies showing that intermittent fasting can help us get rid of cancer once and for all. If you didn't know, there was one man who fasted for ten days Non-Stop and got rid of his disease. We don't know how accurate that is, and please don't put us on it, but this is what people have been saying about intermittent fasting and cancer. Intermittent fasting is indeed the new way to get rid of cancer, as much professional say. Having to control what you eat and when you eat it is essential, what intermittent fasting does is that it allows us to get rid of all the bad cells in our body by using a full cycle known as autophagy. Has General Auto Peggy as a process where your body gets rid of the old battery and makes new cells in your body. This is why intermittent fasting can and will reduce the risk of cancer, consider that when following intermittent fasting.

Reduce insulin resistance:

As you know, intermittent fasting can reduce insulin sensitivity, which is why intermittent fasting has to be followed by many people if they want to see better results. Insulin sensitivity is significant, and being insulin resistant means that you will not be digesting any food that is going into your body. Many people who have diabetes tend to be insulin resistant, controlling this hormone is very important for overall health and longevity. What intermittent fasting does as it does not spike up your insulin randomly, what it gives you as a leveled insulin level product that will help you not only to say healthy but to help you digest food. This is very important when you're following intermittent fasting and trying to live a long healthy life; controlling this hormone wall dictates how well and how many diseases you can avoid in the future. Make sure you use intermittent fasting for the right reasons, meaning taking care of your health and body. There have been many scientific studies showing that intermittent fasting will make you a lot more insulin sensitive, which is something we want as we get older; we become more insulin resistant.

Increase longevity

With all these benefits comes durability, we have been talking about it briefly in this chapter so far. But as you can see, intermittent fasting and definitely help you with longevity and how long you will live. Which is why periodic fasting is one of the most basic eating plans to follow when it comes to overall health and wellness, the truth is that intermittent fasting will not only help you put on muscle and lose body fat, but it will help you to live a longer life overall. Understanding this is very important when it comes to bettering your life, you have to realize that health is not just about looking good and feeling good it is about longevity and how long you stay healthy for. What intermittent fasting provides you with, is the reduction of any diseases, or attracting any conditions and on top of that, giving you the health and body that you want. Intermittent fasting can indeed increase your longevity. In combination with all these benefits, intermittent fasting can genuinely help you understand what life is about. Increase longevity will give you a lot more benefits such as you get older, and you will not have any health complications or minimal; on top of that, you will not be taking any medications or needing any if you follow a healthful eating plan like intermittent fasting.

DNA

Intermittent fasting has been shown to preserve your DNA and to keep it healthy, and we will not get into this topic to genuinely as it has not been backed up by science as much. However, there have been many studies showing that intermittent fasting will help you not only to fight off any hazardous issues with your DNA, but it will help you preserve it. Preserving your DNA is very important, which is why you need to follow intermittent fasting.

Fertility

Intermittent fasting has been shown to increase productivity in men, as the hormone production goes up, so does the fertility. If you are a man looking to improve your sperm count, then there is no better way for you to go about it than to follow intermittent fasting. This will naturally increase your fertility without messing with any medications, and it is always best for you to increase your sperm count through natural means than to take any medications for it, definitely consider intermittent fasting when trying to increase sperm count or to increase fertility. Now there have been some things that intermittent fasting can increase women's fertility as well. However, we will not tell you that it does, for sure, as it has not been backed up yet.

Cell rejuvenation

As you know, intermittent fasting has been very well-known for autophagy, which is a cell rejuvenation process. When it comes to intermittent fasting and cell Rejuvenation, they going hand-in-hand. If you're looking to better your health and detoxify your body fully, then there's no better way to go about it later to follow intermittent fasting. Make sure that you follow intermittent fasting for the right reasons, which means that you're trying to detoxify your body inside and out. Intermittent fasting will not only detoxify your gut, but it will also detoxify yourself the way it functions everything that you can think of intermittent fasting while detoxified. The truth is that, most of the time, humans are spending their time digesting their food. Therefore, they get in no time to detoxify themselves. We need to detoxify your body naturally, and that comes through starvation, which is why intermittent fasting is one of the best ways to not only rejuvenate yourself but to detoxify your body.

Detox

Now that we have extensively talked about cell rejuvenation let's talk about detoxification and how it works and intermittent fasting. When you're fasting, your body does not have to worry about digestion, which is why it is an excellent idea for your body to start detoxifying itself. This is one of the reasons why he will feel a lot cleaner internally when following intermittent fasting. Many people who follow intermittent fasting feel completely detox within 15 days of starting the plan.

Moreover, intermittent fasting will Detox by everything in your body that you can think about, from your nails to your hair to every single cell in your body. Intermittent fasting is a lot more thorough than a green drink detox, which is why periodic fasting is highly recommended by not only fitness experts but doctors these days. Detoxifying your body is significant, and it is similar to getting an oil change in your car. If you want to keep your vehicle nice and to run, then you need to do regular maintenance, which includes oil change, the same thing goes with your body, which is why you need to detoxify your body as often and as thorough as you can.

Reduce stress and inflammation

Intermittent fasting has shown a significant reduction in inflammation. As you know, information causes a lot of many chronic diseases such as Alzheimer's, dementia, obesity, diabetes, and much more. Now, there are many ways that intermittent fasting helps you get rid of inflammation. The first one being autophagy, as you know, intermittent fasting helps you with cell rejuvenation cleans up itself by eating out the old self and rejuvenating them with the newer, stronger ones. If your body does not rejuvenate itself with more new cells, the older ones that have stayed for an extended period can cause inflammation.

As you know, the average diet does not allow for cell rejuvenation to happen; this is where intermittent fasting comes in as it has been proven to help with the process of autophagy. Another way intermittent fasting enables you to get rid of inflammation would be by producing ketones. When you are fasting, your body uses up all the glycogen stores, which makes it start using stored fat for fuel, and when fats are broken down for energy, ketones are produced. One of the most popular ketones in your body will block a part of your immune system, which is responsible for inflammatory disorders. Another way intermittent fasting helps you lower the risk of inflammation is by making you insulin sensitive. When your body becomes insulin resistant, you will be holding much glucose in your bloodstream. More glucose in your blood will create inflammation, and intermittent fasting allows your body to get rid of all the glucose, which helps you reduce inflammation in your body.

Now that we've talked about many ways intermittent fasting enables you to reduce inflammation, let's talk about how intermittent fasting can help you get rid of stress. You see, inflammation and stress go hand in hand. If you have high levels of inflammation, chances are your stress levels are going to be higher. This means that if you lower your inflammation, you will reduce your stress levels, and as you know, fasting helps with better brain function. Intermittent fasting enables you to send better signals to your brain, which would equal a better functioning brain.

When your mind is functioning at its highest peak, your levels of stress dropdown, better brain function will also help you get rid of any stress you might be having, and having overall better health can help you reduce weight. Overall, all the health benefits you get from intermittent fasting will help you get rid of your stress or at least lower it. This means, even if you are not facing pressure, intermittent fasting will help you have a better functioning brain and also help you get rid of any mental fog or anxiety you might be dealing with. What that in mind, always make sure you consult a physician if you are noticing much more stress than you can handle, as it can be something severe and not fixable by intermittent fasting.

Chapter 3: Different Types of Fasting Protocol

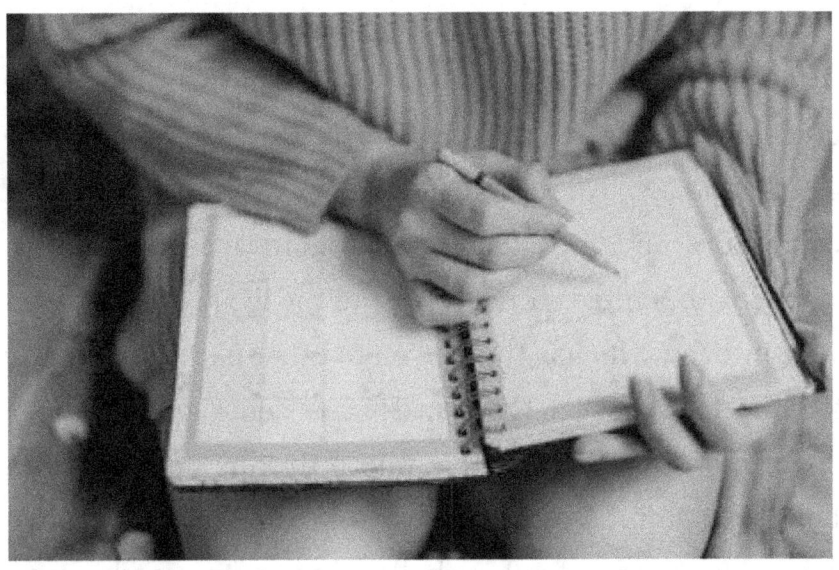

Glucose and fat are the two primary sources of energy for our bodies. Since glucose is more easily broken down than fat, our organization, by default, chooses glucose over fat when both are available. But, if glucose is not possible, the body can quickly turn to fat for its energy needs, and that too, without any harmful effect. At the fundamental level, intermittent fasting compels your body to burn off the excess fat into energy to meet its calorie requirements in the absence of food. What is body fat? It is nothing but excess energy from food that is stored away. If you don't consume, your body will 'eat' the stored fat for its energy needs. Insulin is one of the most critical hormones associated with food digestion.

The level of insulin in your bloodstream increases when you eat. Insulin facilitates the storage of food energy in two ways. First, simple sugars are converted into glycogen and stored in the liver. The liver may have resembled your refrigerator in which it is easy to store and access food, but there is limited space. Second, owing to limited storage space in the liver, glycogen gets converted into fat, which is then taken to other parts of the body and stored as fat deposits. The transfer and deposition of fat is a complex process. But there is no limit on the amount of fat that your body can store. Your body can be compared to a large freezer in which storing food is challenging to store and access. The food stored in that freezer will remain, and if not removed or taken care of, it can turn toxic, just like your fat deposits. The trick in any health-focused regimen, whether it is a diet or fast, is to work on and access the freezer. Therefore, there are two alternative sources of energy in our body.

One is in the form of glycogen (limited amount) in the liver, and the second one is in the way of fat deposits all over the body. The glycogen is easily accessible, whereas the fat is more difficult to access as it is spread all over the body. Now, when the body is in a fasting state, the level of insulin in the blood gets reduced. This reduction in insulin will signal the body to start burning stored energy to meet its energy requirements. The body does not receive food. The glucose level in the blood falls, which means the body will draw stored glycogen from the liver. When this stored glycogen supply is consumed, the body will turn to stored fat for its energy needs. Our organization, therefore, exists in only two states; the fed state where insulin levels are high and the fasting state where insulin levels are low.

In the fed state, our body is storing food energy, and in the fasting state, our body is burning this energy. It's always one state or the other. If we balance the fed and fasting rules, there will be no weight gain. Look at the typical modern-day scenario. We start eating from the minute we get up from sleep in the morning and continue to feed ourselves until we go back to sleep at night. This fed state is continuously storing food energy. There is very little fasting time given to the body to use up this stored energy. Your body will never get an opportunity to burn up the stored energy because you are regularly supplying it with food. There is no balance between the fed and the fasting state resulting in weight gain.

Intermittent fasting helps you regain the essential balance between the fed and the fasting states, thereby helping you lead a healthier life than before. During fasting rules, it is not only fats that are being broken. Realistically, our body uses a combination of lipids (from adipose tissues), ketones (from the fatty acids of the liver), and glucose made from glycogen (in liver and muscles) for its energy during the fasting state. All these forms of energy are needed because different tissues require different kinds of fuel: The muscles use the glucose from the glycogen stored in them for energy or fats from adipose fabrics.

The heart functions excellently with fats. Nerves and the brain prefer to work most efficiently with glucose though they can use ketones too. Red blood cells need only glucose and ketones, or they cannot use fatty acids. Therefore, the body requires to maintain sufficient blood-sugar levels for the RBCs to do their work and for the brain to function correctly. During fasting, this glucose has been converted and stored from the liver into sugar through a process called glycogenolysis. The liver is also capable of converting stored fat and amino acids into glucose. The method of metabolism in our body is quite complicated, and it is essential to remember that it needs all three macronutrients to function efficiently. Fasting empowers our metabolic system to leverage the power of stored fat for nearly all its energy purposes.

Types of Intermittent Fasting

There are various types of intermittent fasting, which is one of the reasons for its flexibility of use. Depending on your suitability, you can choose one or more methods. You could start with the easiest and most popular way, and slowly advance to more complicated options at your pace.

The 12-12 Method

This is the easiest and the most popular method of intermittent fasting and is perfect for beginners. You could already be in this schedule unwittingly. In this method, you have an eating window of 12 hours and a fasting window of 12 hours. So, if your dinner time is 8 pm and you have breakfast the next morning at 8 am, then you are already on this schedule, and you don't even know it. If you have been snacking after dinner, you should stop it immediately. For beginners, this method is excellent to get your body and mind strict about eating and feasting windows.

The 16:8

Method This is also achievable by most novices. However, it can be a massive challenge for people who don't like to miss dinner

AND breakfast. The keyword here is 'AND.' For this method to be a success, you must be ready to skip one of these two meals. By skipping one of the two flours, you will get a 16-hour fasting window, which includes your 8-hour sleeping time. Your feeding window will be a balance of 8 hours a day. For people who have never fasted before, this method could be a high starting point. Finish your dinner by 8 pm and get to bed by 10 pm. When you wake up at 6 am the next morning, 10 hours of the fasting period is already done. Skip breakfast, and you can have your first meal of the day at noon. Just make sure you hydrate yourself well during the fasting window.

Also, you can drink tea or coffee, black and sugarless, which can help fight hunger pangs. Although initially, it might be tough, it does get more comfortable as you persist. During the feasting window, you can fit in 2 or 3 meals. This method is referred to as the Leangains protocol and was made accessible by Martin Berkhan, a famous fitness expert. The dinner-skipping way of following the Leangains process involves an eating window from 8 am – 4 pm (your last meal of the day) and a fasting window of 4 pm – 8 am the next day. If 4 pm for your previous lunch is very far away from your bedtime, you can shift your eating to 10 am (your first meal of the day) to 6 pm (your last meal of the day). Here is a small chart to help you understand how you can plan your 16:8 daily intermittent fasting schedules: If your first meal is at 7 AM, your last meal should be at 3 pm. If your first meal is at 8 AM, your last meal should be at 4 pm. If your first meal is at 11 AM, your last meal should be at 7 pm. If your first meal is at 2 PM, your last meal should be at 10 pm. The 18:6 Method This method will test your willpower a little more than the 16:8 process. It is more challenging to achieve than the previous way as you need to gather all your mental strength and fight off hunger pangs for 18 hours; 2 hours more than 16! Moreover, with an eating window of only 6 hours, you cannot get more than two meals, and perhaps, squeeze in one little snack in-between. The good thing about this method is once you have perfected it and your body and mind have come to accept it as part of your life, you don't have to try any more extreme intermittent fasting methods.

The 18:6 method

Will suffice for the rest of your life. You can extend each day's fasting regimen to cover more hours for fasting and lesser hours for eating. For example, you could have a fasting window for 20 hours and an eating window of 4 hours (20:4, tough yes, but doable over a long period). Or, you could have one meal a day in which you ensure you get all the nutrients your body needs. The last two methods are extreme and cannot be done daily. You can keep them for special days to test your mental strength and willpower capacity. Even the keenest fasting advocates might not be able to manage the 20:4 and one-meal-a-day consistently. Additionally, any extreme fasting method to be maintained for more than a couple of days should never be attempted without medical supervision.

The 5:2 Diet

This method of intermittent fasting entails following a healthy eating pattern (without any fasting schedule) on five days of the week and restricting calorie intake to 500-600 calories on two days. This diet is called the Fast Diet and was made famous by Michael Mosley, a British doctor, and journalist. Women are advised to consume 500 calories and men 600 calories on the two fasting days of the week. A great example of the 5:2 diet would be to restrict calorie intake on Mondays and Thursdays, and generally eating on all the other days. You can choose any two days that are suitable for you. However, the most effective way of doing this fast is to choose two consecutive fasting days when you will restrict your calorie intake to 500-600. Your metabolism will highly benefit from this method of fasting, especially if you can manage two consecutive fasting days instead of two separate days.

The 24-Hour Fast

While eating one meal a day regularly is not just difficult but also not highly advised, fasting one day a week for 24 hours is doable and a great intermittent fasting method too. Brad Pilon, another famous fitness expert, advocated and popularized this method of intermittent fasting. Dinner at 7 pm on Monday, followed by dinner at 7 pm on Tuesday, is an example of the 24-hour fasting method. You could also choose to do breakfast-to-breakfast or lunch-to-lunch. During the 24-hour fasting period, only tea, coffee, and other non-calorie liquids are allowed. The trick to making a success of this intermittent fasting method is to stick to generally eating on your first meal after the 24-hour fasting period. You must consume the same amount of food that you would have eaten had you not fasted. Again, staying in the fasting mode for 24 hours can be a considerable challenge for many. The first few hours might go off uneventfully, but later on, ravenous hunger can create a lot of temporary discomforts. You will have to give your best self-discipline ways to make this method a success. However, you don't need to start in such a rigorous way. Instead of starting at the 24-hour level, you can begin with a 14-16-hour level on one day of the first week, and slowly increase it to 24 hours after 3-4 weeks or at your pace. The Alternate-Day Fasting Method This method requires you to fast every other day and usually eat every other day. On the fasting days, your calorie intake should be restricted to 500-600. The alternate-day fasting method calls for going hungry to bed several days each week, which may not be an easy or pleasant thing to do and can be quite an extreme method.

The Warrior Diet

This method of intermittent fasting entails consuming: Fruits and raw vegetables in small quantities during the day. One big meal at dinner time. Primarily, the warrior diet consists of fasting all day and feasting at one feast. However, it is different from the rigorous 24-hour fasting diet because here, you do consume fruits and vegetables, which can be great to stave off hunger pangs effectively and in a healthy manner.

The nighttime meal is typically similar to the paleo diet consisting of wholesome and unprocessed foods that are as close to how nature provides them as possible. Despite the fruits and vegetables, the Warrior Diet can be quite a challenge. As beginners, it might not make sense to try it until you have understood how your body responds to more straightforward methods of intermittent fasting. Spontaneous Intermitting Fasting This method does not have any structure or planning for it. You choose to skip one or two meals if you are not feeling hungry or do not have the time to cook, or you feel like it or for any other reason.

Having to eat regularly to remain energized and active is nothing but a myth. The fear of entering 'starvation mode' looms so large that we end up eating far more than what we need. Our body is well-equipped to manage not just missing a couple of meals but times of great famine. So, if you do not feel hungry, don't hesitate to skip a couple of meals. Just be conscious of not overeating when you do sit down to your meal after a couple of skips. Also, stick to healthy foods during your mealtimes. The trick in intermittent fasting is to cut calorie intake by cutting down the number of meals. Skipping meals whenever you feel inclined is referred to as spontaneous intermitting fasting. The flip side of this method is a lack of plan and strategy that could lead you to become irreverent and undisciplined in your approach leading to ineffective results. However, if you are a naturally disciplined person and have ingrained the habit of intermittent fasting into your system, then the spontaneous method will work correctly.

The water fast

Well, the name says it all; this method has got to be one most laborious fasting methods that you can follow. Most of the ways can be used for an extended period, but I would suggest this method is only used only certain times a year. I would only use this method as a tool rather than a lifestyle, as doing this for too long can do some damage to your body. That being said, this method can be used to your advantage, but first, let's talk about how this method works.

This method is based on you eating like you usually would, and then fasting for one to three days with the only thing that you can have during your fasting period is water. The best way to start this fast is to plan it ahead of time, slowly lower the calories every day as you get closer to your pool fast as it will prepare your body, and it won't be such a shock. An example will be if you were consuming two thousand calories day, what I would recommend is to lower five hundred calories every day, so on the fourth day, you can start your fast without it being a shock. Now the best way to go about fasting is to fast for one to two days no longer than three days, some people have fasted for ten days using this method, but I would not recommend you go without food for that long, and I don't see the reason why you should be fasting for so long. Since there are not a lot of guidelines on how often should you fast using this method, the best way would be to use this method is to fast every four to eight weeks, and I wouldn't go past three days of actual fasting. I would recommend you fast on days that you are not doing anything physically like working out since it can affect your workout and your whole day after that. One thing I would recommend you don't do is to use this method more than twelve times in a year, as doing it often can affect your day to day life and energy levels based on experiences. Although this method can't be used as a lifestyle, there are some benefits to these methods, so let's talk about them.

This method is best known for cleaning out toxins in your body. Since you won't eat for one to three days and the only thing that you will be consuming is water, your body will automatically get rid of toxins in your body with the help of water. This has got be a selling point for me when it comes to using this method, don't get me wrong every fasting method helps with cleaning out your body, but if your body doesn't ingest anything for one to three days, then that gives your body plenty of time to "clean up." Another fantastic benefit of using this method is that it will clean out any harmful bacteria in your gut, which will help you digest your food better the next time you consume some. Since you will be getting rid of toxins in your body, you will also get the benefit of lowered risk of diseases, which is always a plus. Another thing this method can help you with is a fat loss since you won't be eating for so long your body will depend on fat for energy, but I would not use this method for fat loss as there are other methods that you can use for that goal. As you can see, this method has some benefit, now let us talk about some issues that you can have with this method.

The first issue with this method is that it can be super hard to go thru with. Fasting for one to three days with no food requires a lot of will power, and often, people won't go thru with this method since it's so hard. Another issue that this method could have is that it can affect your strength, if you are into strength training then be prepared to lose some strength following this plan to often, This issues can be kept in control if you fast on non-workout days and use this method every four to eight weeks. One of the major flaws with this method is that there is a chance that you can go hypoglycemic, so be careful as this can get super dangerous if you fast for an extended period. These are the main issues with using this method, most of the problems can be fixed if you be careful and don't use this method often meaning not exceeding more than three days of fasting and easing into the technique.

The Positives of Intermittent

Fasting If you plan your meals to fit into a smaller eating window, you are more likely to be a conscious eater than if you choose to leave the entire day open to eat whenever you like. With intermittent fasting, you tend to become a more mindful eater than before. Eating mindlessly is one of the biggest causes of binge-eating. Another thing about intermittent fasting is that while you have to keep a general control over calorie intake, you don't have to micromanage this aspect.

Therefore, given the freedom to eat what you want (in reasonable amounts) could drive you to consume healthier foods. Many times, excessive restrictions encourage us to do something we should not do. Intermittent fasting gives you a reasonable amount of freedom to eat your favorite foods during your eating window. The Negatives of Intermittent Fasting For some people, the fact that you can eat whatever you want can be counterproductive because they end up binge-eating at every meal during the eating window. This approach will end up defeating the core desire of intermittent fasting, and you could eat far more than needed resulting in weight gain and an unhealthy lifestyle.

The initial hiccups could drive some people to overreact to hunger pangs and cravings, resulting in cultivating worse eating habits than before. All the initial setbacks of intermittent fasting and how to cope with them are discussed in greater detail. Moreover, restricting the time of eating could also make some people think that it is another form of 'diet.' This dieting mindset can be detrimental to achieving your intermittent fasting goals. A necessary mindset of 'following a diet' will make you less likely to follow through the process than you look at it as an altered eating pattern. The most important thing you must remember about intermittent fasting is that it is not a crash diet that you can try for 3-5 days before an upcoming party to fit into a dress you've bought for yourself. It is a choice of a lifetime to change the way you eat for the rest of your life. Read on for more benefits, cautionary advice, and more about intermittent fasting.

Chapter 4: How to Pick the Right Plan Based on Your Lifestyle

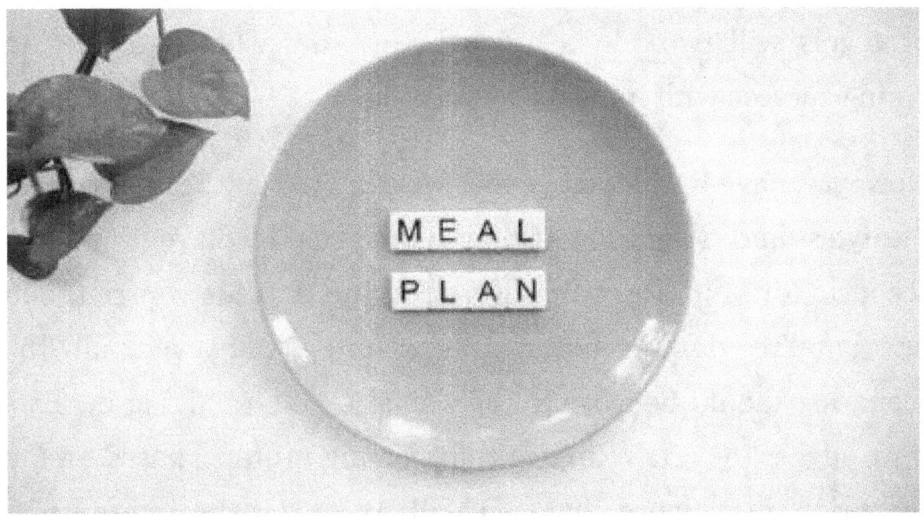

In this chapter, we will help you understand how to pick out the right plan when it comes to intermittent fasting protocol. One thing to realize would be that intimate fasting can be customized based on your needs. If you are someone looking to have eating schedules based on your lifestyle, then chances are intermittent fasting is the answer for you. As you know, by now, there are tons of ways for you to follow intermittent fasting. We talked about the different intermittent fasting protocols, and which one will benefit you in what way. One thing to remember is that you will still see many of the benefits we discussed in the previous chapters, regardless of the plan you follow. Which means that following intermittent fasting or certain protocol should not demotivate you when it comes to following a certain plan. With that being said, what we will do in this chapter is it go through different Lifestyles and how certain intermittent fasting protocols will work in a much better way when it comes to seeing success with intermittent fasting.

Now, you have to remember that we can only go through certain lifestyles and scenarios. Don't expect us to have a perfect scenario for you. You will have to decide that for yourself, and once you're done reading this chapter. However, all the scenarios should be close to the scenario you are living in. also, if we suggest a certain intermittent fasting protocol based on the scenarios, make sure that you still try on all the intermittent fasting protocols and realize which one works for you. The truth is, the best personal trainer is the best nutritionist you're going to have you. Once you start understanding your body, then you will be in a much better position of not only utilizing intermittent fasting at its full potential, but you also have a great idea off went to stop and when you should begin.

If that makes sense, then you should be steps ahead of your trainers and nutritionists, which you might hire. We are not saying that you should not have a personal trainer or nutritionist, what we are saying is that you will be in a much better position if you can understand how your body functions to create a customized plan for you. Now the first scenario we are going to be using would be very similar to someone who works in a nine-to-five job. If your someone who works from 9 to 5 and only gets one lunch break during the day and chances are 16/ 8, intermittent fasting would be ideal for you. To clarify, you can always start with a 12/12 intermittent fasting protocol, in the beginning, to get ready. However, once you get your feet wet with intermittent fasting, then you should go with the 16/8 method.

The reason why the 16/8 method works so well for people who work a 9to five job it is because it is straightforward to manage. The beauty of the 16/8 method when it comes to intermittent fasting is that you can set the hours to whatever time you want to eat, and you don't want to eat. For example, many people notice better brain functioning when they are not eating any food. This means you can skip breakfast and not eat throughout the whole workday allowing you to focus on the task at hand. Then once you're done working, you can have yourself a nice big breakfast. We know numerous amounts of people doing this, and not only did the notice they lost a lot of weight, but they also got a lot better at the work which they are performing. The beauty of intermittent fasting would be that it allows you to not only lose body fat but give you the mental clarity that you're looking for.

The reason why you get mental Clarity is that you will not be spiking up your insulin throughout the day. When you spike up your insulin, you will notice things such as lethargy and overall laziness. This is why the 16/8 method works so great when it comes to recovering any issues which you might be facing when it comes to mental fog or mental fatigue. That being said, start with the 12/12 method and slowly build-up to the 16/8 method to see better results. In this scenario, not only will your work performance go up, but you also lose a lot of weight and get the overall health benefit that you're looking for when it comes to intermittent fasting. This will work especially well for people who are above the age of 50.

The reason why it will work a lot better for people who are above the age of 50 is simply that they will go through a phase known as autophagy. As you know, autophagy has been shown to reduce many health complications, including the slowing down of aging. This makes it ideal for people looking to slow down aging. So if you work a nine-to-five job and you're looking to lose body fat while slowing down aging, then we highly recommend that you follow the 16/8 method throughout the workday. Meaning fastest route to the workday, and have yourself a nice breakfast after you're done working. I want you to perform a lot better at your workplace, and to see better results overall when it comes to intermittent fasting and losing body fat. Keep in mind, the scenario we just talked about is the first scenario that most people will be going through.

However, we have a ton of scenarios to talk about. now chances are there will be a lot of people who work in labor, looking to reap the benefits of intermittent fasting. Now, if you are working labor, chances are it will be a little bit more difficult for you to continue with intermittent passing. However, with the right scheduling in the right planning, you should have no problem concerning intermittent fasting. now let's say you work the labor 8 hours a day. What we would recommend is trying to have most of your calories throughout the 8-hour window. Once you are done with your work, make sure that you start your fast right away.

Now there are a lot of ways for you to get your calories throughout your eating window while you are working. You can have things such as protein shake, and You are quickly you going to have a pre-prepared meal, which will help you to consume all the calories you need throughout the whole day. The reason why we recommend you eat throughout the day while you're working is that a labor job could be tedious. We want to make sure that you don't paint or affect your work in any way possible. This is why we recommend you follow the 16 by eight method and include your eating window while you are working. Many people who work in labor tend to follow this protocol, the reason why it works so well. That's because they won't get all the calories they need when they need it. you need to have a good steady flow of food intake while you are physically working.

Your body can only break down fat so quickly, which is why a good amount of carbohydrates and nutrients is important when you're performing anything physical. That being said, you can always resort to the 5/2 method when you are intermittent fasting. If you don't like the 16/8 method, then you can always follow the 5/2 method. This method works great as you only have to "fast" for two days out of the week, meaning you can normally eat when you are working. As you get older, especially in the labor workforce, you will be required to be well-fed when you're working. The last thing we want is for you to have injuries at your workplace. That being said, you can either follow the 16/8 method, or you can go right ahead and follow the 5/2 method fasting on your non-working days.

This will allow you to see the results that you're looking for when it comes to anti-aging, regardless of the fasting protocol you follow. However, if we're honest, the 16/8 method works a lot better when it comes to seeing results in regards to intermittent fasting and anti-aging. Now let's pick out another scenario, what's talked about someone who works the night shift. If you're someone who works the night shift, the chances are that you will be in a much better scenario than a lot of people. The reason why you will be in a much better position than a lot of people is that nightshift tends to be slow for most cases. Now, if you're a nurse, then chances are you will have no time to eat any food.

So the best thing for you to do would be not to have any food during your shift, and once you're done your shift, you can have more food allowing you to be a lot better at fasting. The great thing about being a nurse or working a night shift would be that you will have a much better position of not only continued with intermittent fasting but the desire to not eat. Numerous times we have heard nurses talk about not having the time to eat, or simply not in the mood for eating anything. Having this mentality will help you tremendously to continue with intermittent fasting, which is why it is so important to understand which intermittent fasting protocol works for your needs. Batting said if your nurse is working night shifts, the best-case scenario for you would be too fast brought your whole shift and have your eating window once you're done your work. For instance, let's say you work 10 hours a day, then fast for 10 hours a day and eat for the remainder of the time. This gets a little bit tricky for a nurse, as the hours can be scattered or sometimes not be ideal case scenario for you too fast. However, the best way to go about fasting if your nurse who is who works a shift at a very demanding job, we recommend you fast during the time you are working. This will allow you to be in a perfect position when it comes to fasting and to see the best results overall with intermittent fasting. In essence, you will be trying out all the types of intermittent fasting when you are working the night shift or working as a nurse, for example. Depending on your shift, you will be fasting either 10 hours or even up to 24 hours, depending on how you feel. That being said, this will give you the best possible scenario for you to continue with intermittent fasting and to make it a habit. Many people don't realize it, but making intermittent fasting a part of your life is much more important than someone looking to follow a specific plan. Now we have given you enough scenarios to figure out which plan would work best for you based on your lifestyle. Now we will move on and talk about all the methods and which deliver the specific goal that you're looking for. Keep in mind that all these plans will work tremendously well if you're looking to slow down aging and to lose body fat overall feeling better about yourself. However, we will break down all the plans so that you have a better idea of which one to pick and finalize.

16/8: As you know, the 16/8 method is one of the most popular ways when it comes to intermittent fasting. The 16/8 way will not only help you to lose body fat, but it will also help you with the anti-aging process and to better your overall function. Many people follow the 16/8 method as it is the most convenient method to follow and comfortably flexible. Depending on your lifestyle, this method could work very well when it comes to giving you the results that you're looking for. The beauty of this method is that you can build muscle, lose fat, and do anything you want while making this a life choice. When I say a life choice, it means that you can follow this plan for the rest of your life and not feel taxed out. If it is feasible for you, then we highly recommend that you follow the 16/8 method, one of the most studied ways of intermittent fasting.

12/12: Now, this method is for someone who's looking to set up intermittent fasting without going too hard if you don't know how intermittent fasting works or you don't know if it is going to be the right path for you then you should start with the 12/12 method. This method will allow you to get your feet wet when it comes to intermittent fasting so that you can continue with intermittent fasting if you enjoy it or make it a little bit more challenging by upping the fasting times. That being said, but 12/12 method is merely something to get your feet wet with and not something you should do for the rest of your life. The secure trolls method is a great plan to start. However, you will not see the anti-aging effects or the weight loss effects that you're looking for following this method. In the beginning, you will, however, as you go along, you will not see the results that you are looking for when it comes to losing body fat are slowing down the aging process. This is where the 16/8 method will shine, as it will give you sufficient time to fast while seeing the benefits that you are hoping to get out of intermittent fasting.

The water fast: Now the water fast is for someone who is looking to not only detoxify their body, but they're changing the way their body functions. This plan is only to be followed a handful of times to detoxify their gut, so they digest a lot better. If you might know, the stomach is known as the second brain. The reason why it is known as a second brain is that your body heavily depends on your gut and how it digests, as you know, eating food as necessary for a livelihood, which is why we must take care of the organs, especially our gut. Make sure you use this method to clean out your organs and to see better results from it. This will allow you to be in a better position when it comes to digesting food and keeping your organs beautiful and safe.

5:2 Diet: This fasting protocol is ideal for people who are looking to lose weight quickly, now if you're someone who wants to lose weight rapidly and has a motivation and willpower to get it done then the 5/2 works the best. A disciple makes you lose a lot of body fat and a short period, allowing you to live a lot better life overall. Now keep in mind that following the 5/2 diet will not help you with any anti-aging process in the long-term. But I will help you detoxify your body and to make you lose a ton of weight, especially in the beginning. Don't follow this protocol for the rest of your life as it is not sustainable. However, once you get the hang of this plan, you will be in a much better position to lose fat and to get your goal weight a lot quicker than you would.

Once you've lost a way to find the 5/2 diet, we recommend that you started following the 16/8 diet quickly. The 16/8 diet is where you want to be when it comes to seeing long-lasting results. Regardless of the 5/2 diet will work for you if you do a labor job, because of the structure.

This chapter should give you a clear idea of how intermittent fasting works and which protocol you should be following when it comes to bettering your results based on your lifestyle. Now some people might find this chapter very basic or vague. Keep in mind that we want you to use your brain when it comes to picking out the right plan. If you remember in the beginning, we told you that the best nutritionist or the trainer for you would be yourself, which is why we need you to understand this chapter and pick up the plan which works for your lifestyle and your goals. As always, make sure that you know your body before you start following any of these plans. We recommend a start off with a 12/12 method as you will see significant benefits from it in the beginning. However, once you get your feet wet with intermittent fasting, then we recommend that you start following other plans that will help you achieve that goal as well.

Chapter 5: How Does Intermittent Fasting Slow Down Aging

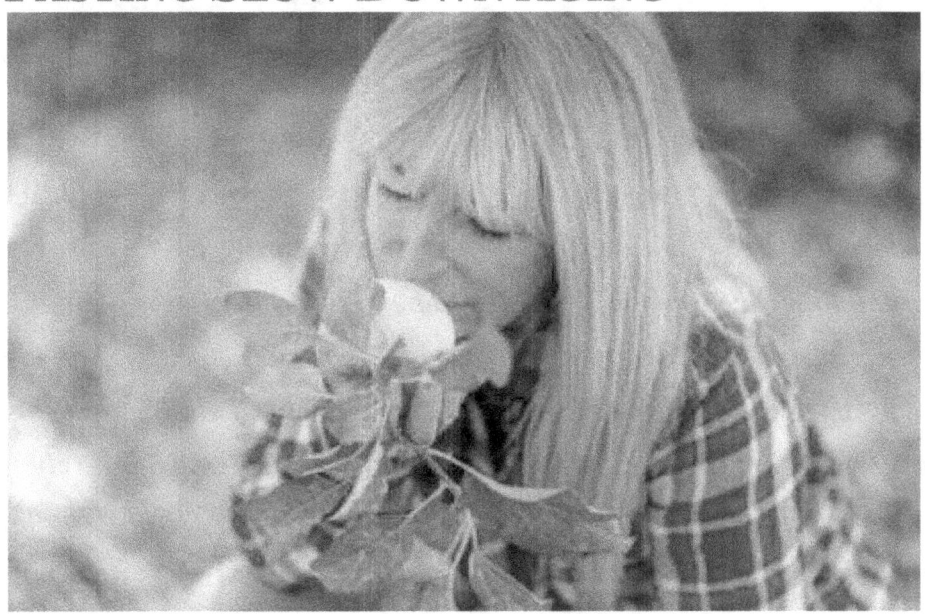

When we were kids, it sometimes felt like we couldn't wait to grow up, so we didn't have to listen to our parents. Even when we graduated high school, we might have wished we could be even older so we could drink alcohol, have a better job, and just more freedom in general. Once you hit a certain age, you start to realize that as you get older time goes by faster each year as well. Not only this, but it's harder to keep up with your health. You might have been able to eat nothing but potato chips and ice cream in a day and felt fine, but that same kind of meal now could sound like a night of indigestion. We can never reverse aging, and until we have a time machine, there's no going back. You will always be as old as you've ever been, and as young as you will ever be, the rest of your life, each moment that you live. This kind of thinking can be terrifying, but it's also important to remember as we choose the right type of diets for our health. The better choices you make, the longer your life can be. There will always be certain unavoidable things and accidents which can change our plans, however, that doesn't mean we shouldn't be trying to live as long as possible, as healthy as we can be. *Reducing the Stress Hormone Levels: An increase in insulin levels can also be directly affected by our stress levels. When we feel stressed out, our bodies release cortisol. This hormone is necessary to provide energy to our muscular system. When you're stressed, your body will go into a flight/fight mode, which helps protect you against this threat felt. This is why you might notice your shoulders are sore when you're stressed, or that you keep your jaw and fists clenched, resulting in some muscle fatigue. This release of cortisol can also mean a higher level of glucose throughout your bloodstream. If you are stressed out all the time, then this means you are continually releasing that cortisol, steadily increasing your blood sugar. Stress that results in no physical activity isn't good either, because then you're just holding onto that energy. If we want to reduce our insulin levels and keep our body regulated, then stress needs to be managed as well* (Kresser, 2019).

Lowering the Insulin Levels As you get older, it's harder to keep up with your health. Even those who actively try to eat healthily and the workout will find that they struggle a lot more in their older years than they did when they were young and healthy teens. Those at any age who eat unhealthily are at risk of forming insulin resistance and certain types of diabetes. Diabetes is much more common in older individuals, meaning if we want to keep our health long throughout our lives, we need to focus on regulating insulin right now. We already discussed how fasting could control your insulin and keep you from becoming insulin resistant, so no need to explain that again here.

What's important to remember, however, is that you should always consider an increase in your insulin sensitivity as you get older. It's not easy to accept, but our health will only get more challenging to manage, so we need to focus on doing that now so we can live a long and happy life. Keeping Your Liver Healthy One thing we haven't talked about, yet very much is your liver, and how this can affect your health. You might instantly think about alcohol when it comes to your liver, knowing that too much alcohol can have adverse effects on this. However, your liver is responsible for a lot more than just processing the alcohol you drink. A detox of your liver can help in your process of losing weight. However, after you've gone through rehab, then you need to keep up with a healthy lifestyle, or else your liver will be subjected to the same things. The thing about your liver is that this is the part of your body that helps detoxify! It is your body's filtration system, helping to remove toxins throughout your body. While it is mighty and even capable of regenerating itself, you still need to treat it right, giving it as few toxins to get rid of as possible. The first toxin that you will run into is additives to any processed foods. This is going to include things like food dyes and artificial flavors that aren't typically meant for regular consumption.

Alternatively, consider other chemicals, pesticides, and hormones that are added to processed foods, which could directly affect the efficiency of your liver. Intermittent fasting is an excellent choice for your liver because it is a process to detox your body. Think of it like giving your liver a little break from its job. As you process fatty stored cells during a fast, these are simple things already broken down once in your body, meaning that when your liver does have to do work, it will be easier than what it might have been subjected to in the past. As we get older, we'll start to get more sensitive to other kinds of illnesses, meaning our filtration system will need to improve. There's no better time to start taking care of your liver than now (Browning, 2012). How to Use Fasting for Longevity Fasting promotes a healthier lifestyle and encourages better habits. Since it is a natural way to lose weight, it will last you longer. You could try out a complicated diet involving meal replacements and supplements, but at the end of the day, this might result in you gaining weight faster than you lost it. The fluctuation of weight gain and loss isn't always right on our bodies. To live a long and healthy life, you have to make healthy choices. Train your body to burn fat and detoxify continually, and you will be doing your very best to try and achieve longevity through the use of fasting.

Autophagy is when cells can clean themselves. It involves the process of a cell removing the toxins and other unwanted substances that might have penetrated their makeup. This would need to be done when a virus, harmful bacteria, or other poison has made its way into the body, regardless of the type of intruder versus cell attacked (Murrell, 2018). Whenever a foreign particle might be present, then your cells will be able to fight that or remove it using autophagy. Autophagy occurs throughout the day without us having any idea what's happening. Your body is smart, so just because you're adding things to it that are damaging doesn't mean that it's always going to feel those effects.

Our bodies aren't perfect, however, so they will still need some help through other processes that can kickstart or encourage autophagy. *Cleaning of Waste Cells and Pathogens: The stronger the cell, the better it will be able to clean waste and get rid of various pathogens in the body. Fasting is a great way to encourage autophagy and cause your cells to not only rid themselves of toxins but to repair new, stronger ones as well* (Murrell, 2018). You might notice some detoxes are doing things aimed at specific detoxification, such as a liver detox, a heart detox, or even a brain detox. This isn't necessary, as encouraging autophagy throughout your body will help work to clean it starting from the inside and eventually spreading throughout your body. *Stop Progression of Diseases: Autophagy could even help encourage the reduction of cancer cells, or at least help to prevent them from growing in the first place* (Bhutia, 2013). We have numerous mitochondria throughout our bodies that get older with time. Once they get to a certain age, they will start to release free radicals in our collection. These could end up causing mutations, sometimes mortal. To produce new mitochondria and rid ourselves of the old, then we will need to focus on encouraging autophagy within our bodies. Caloric restriction is the best way to reduce this at first. This isn't a cure-all, but caloric restriction has been helped to slow down the production and growth of various tumors (Murrell, 2018). This can be very specific, so you mustn't assume fasting is going to cure cancer. It might help prevent and reduce, but it's not necessarily a cure-all. To avoid it in the first place, encourage autophagy within your cells.

How Autophagy Impacts You

Autophagy will have many other benefits to your health that are important to understand. It helps with reducing the amount of stored fat, which is a benefit in itself while also helping to prevent other health conditions associated with being overweight. It can help repair damaged cells, which is essential to keep up productivity from where those cells are damaged. For example, if some cells in your stomach are damaged from a life of unhealthy eating, autophagy could help to repair those. All of this will also help reduce inflammation, which can have other serious health risks as well. When you experience redness, it can slow down specific processes and cause your organs to not work as well, depending on where the inflammation is present.

When you get a cut, it turns red and swells – this is inflammation. When we damage our bodies inside, they will become inflamed; we won't see it. This could have adverse health effects, such as sore and tight joints, slow-working systems (such as a digestive system that isn't working correctly/causes pain to use), and could even cause depression through an inflamed brain (Raison, 2011). If you don't have autophagy within your body's function, it puts you at risk for some cardiovascular, rheumatological, atherosclerosis, and pulmonary diseases. You might also be at a higher risk of cancer, holding onto more fat, muscle loss, and even sensitivity to the sun. Protein Cycling One way to induce autophagy is to use protein cycling. This is the process of having some higher amounts of protein during some phases and lowers at others. When fasting, it will be best to reduce your protein intake on the days that you are restricting your food. On your days of eating and no fasting, then you can go back to a reasonable amount of protein. Fasting days stick to 25 grams or less.

Other days, you can go back to normal, which is 46-56 grams depending on your sex/body weight. The point of keeping yourself from overeating protein will be to force your body to look elsewhere for its energy source. When Autophagy and Protein Cycling Matter Especially for Women These processes are essential to include even in those that don't want to lose weight because autophagy will reduce over time and become less efficient as we get older. This is especially important for women because we are at risk for certain estrogen-related diseases and cancers, and we usually have a higher fat content than the average healthy man. We want autophagy to work for us, and to reduce our body's toxins continually, so ensure that you are regulating your autophagy effectiveness through intermittent fasting. We already know by now that fasting will make your cells turn on themselves, fat being burned along the process.

Autophagy is your body's natural way of doing this, so it's clear to see that incorporating fasting will help to kickstart that natural process that already exists. Autophagy occurs within the first 24 hours of fasting, on average. This means that you aren't fasting for 24-hours, but you've restricted your caloric intake.

How to Induce Autophagy Through Intermittent Fasting

You might see supplements, teas, or other products that claim they induce autophagy. Still, the only obvious way that's proven to be safe and effective is to do it naturally through fasting. As you fast, you are lowering your insulin levels. Therefore, you have a higher chance of starting autophagy within your body. What's most important to induce autophagy is focusing on reducing your glycogen levels, which only shows after around 14 hours of fasting. For longer health, you will want to include extended periods of fasting for weeks, but preferably, months, at a time.

Chapter 6: How Should Women Fast Over 50?

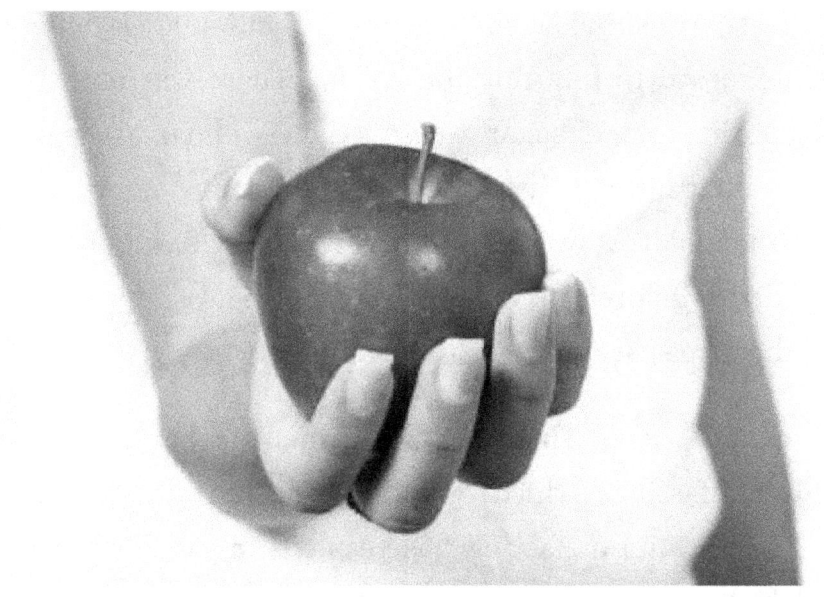

As we mentioned to you previously, intermittent fasting does not yield drastically different results in both men and women. However, there are many differences in regard to how women should follow intermittent fasting. The great news is that women can take part in all the fast's listed in this book, regardless we need to talk about intermittent fasting for women.

Some claims are suggesting that intermittent fasting needs to be modified, which is true to a certain degree if women use the easier going fasting protocols, which are available to review in the previous chapters. Then they should have no problem with intermittent fasting, and the problems start to occur when 48 hours+ fasts begin to take place.

Nonetheless, you should know the claims and studies done on women in regard to intermittent fasting. There was one study suggesting that blood sugar worsened in women after three weeks of intermittent fasting. Moreover, many sources are claiming that changes in women's menstrual cycle will occur. As we explained before, because of the woman's reproductive system, they are susceptible to lower calories.

Hence, making people believe that women do not indulge in intermittent fasting, which we don't agree with. If done tastefully, intermittent fasting has resulted in excellent health and weight loss benefits for women. So in this chapter, we will go thru exactly how occasional fasting affects women in all aspects, such as hormones, hunger craving, and many more things are on the agenda. With that in mind, let's get into the nitty-gritty.

The key to intermittent fasting for women in autophagy

You might have heard of autophagy in this book so far, now let me explain to you what autophagy truly means. Autophagy is a biological process that comes to the Greek word "auto," meaning "self" and "phagy," meaning "eat." It is a process where our body cleans out the bad cells and replace them with newer healthy ones, which is excellent for anyone looking to live a healthier life.

But sometimes, our body cannot get this process going for hosts of reasons. Mainly because we eat the food we can't digest properly, which makes our body work extra hard to cope up with the food instead of getting rid of "bad cells." As we get older, the process becomes less efficient. One of the proven ways to fix this issue, especially for women, is by fasting for 12 or more hours and allowing your body to focus more on getting rid of the "bad cells" by replacing them with newer and stronger ones.

This method works exceptionally well, especially on women, to rejuvenate their cells and to see the health benefits. The great news about autophagy is that you don't need to fast for an indefinite amount of time to notice the results, 12 to 16 hours of fast will do. This means women don't need to put yourself at risk by fasting for a prolonged period; this makes intermittent fasting a tool for women looking to stay young for more extended periods.

Remember that autophagy should not be just for anti-aging purposes, as it can help you with hosts of things. Consider autophagy as a detox for your whole body, and believe it or not; most people need it. Forget cleansing diets, and if you truly want to detox your body, then you need to fast for at least 12 hours a day.

For women, 12-16 hours should not result in adverse effects. You will also reduce the risk of cancer because you will have newer and stronger cells at your disposal; another great benefit would be the fact that your metabolism will go up helping you with weight loss.

All in all, promoting the process of autophagy a great way to encourage better health, especially for women. Having healthier cells in a women's body will help you by having a better reproductive system, and you will have a higher chance of conceiving. Even though these claims haven't been backed up, it is still good to know that some excellent benefits come with intermittent fasting for women.

Finally, you will notice benefits such as better skin, better digestion of more energy throughout the day. To see the best results, fast for 12 to 16 hours a day, three times a week. Make sure you space out your days, instead of doing all the fasts back to back. If you want to fast through the week as many do, then make sure not to prolong it for more than 6-8 weeks.

Fasting and female hormones

Intermittent fasting has shown to affect females' hormones, and there are some things women need to consider before they start fasting. Some studies are showing how intermittent fasting can negatively impact the female's reproductive system, and the reason why these shifts occur is that women are sensitive to lower calorie intake. When the calories are low for women, a small part of the brain known as the hypothalamus is affected.

Hypothalamus can disrupt the production of gonadotropin-releasing hormone (GnRH), which is responsible for releasing the two reproductive hormones, luteinizing hormone (LH) and follicle-stimulating hormone (FSH). Once these hormones have been affected negatively from an extended period by restricting calories, you will be running a risk of irregular periods, infertility, poor bone health, and other health risks. Even though autophagy has shown to do the opposite, it puts women in a complicated situation when it comes to fasting. For that reason, we don't recommend women fast for more than 24 hours as it can affect women's hormones in a very drastic manner.

Instead, women should use a modified approach that we talked about in this book. To make sure women don't notice any hormone imbalance, fast alternate days instead of back to back, keeping you in a safe place. If you want to fast aggressively for weight loss, then our recommendation is not to prolong it for more than 4-6 weeks. But then again, make sure you consult a professional before you may start fasting as everybody is different. On the plus side, there are many benefits women will notice if they begin fasting the right way. As we know, heart disease is killing people every day, in one study done on obese women showed that intermittent fasting lowered LDL cholesterol or which is the leading cause of heart problems in North America.

Also, intermittent fasting has shown to make you more insulin sensitive. In one study of 100 obese women showed that six months of intermittent fasting reduced insulin levels by 29% and insulin resistance by 19 %, although blood sugar remained the same. Having higher sensitively to insulin has shown to lower the risk of type 2 diabetes. Still, intermittent fasting may not be beneficial for women as it is for men in regards to blood sugar. In mice, it has been shown to increase longevity by 33%, although long term studies on humans are yet to be determined.

Finally, intermittent fasting can reduce inflammation levels. Even though more studies need to be executed for women and intermittent fasting, it is pretty clear that there are hosts of benefits if done right. As long as you are taking intermittent fasting the right way, and you are not abusing it, your hormones should be in check. Remember, if you are pregnant, this might affect you very differently. Moreover, we do not recommend women fast when they are pregnant or trying to conceive, but as long as you know the repercussions of fasting too long.

Why intermittent fasting affects women's hormones more than men's?

If you have been doing research online, then you might have read claims such as "intermittent fasting is not for women" or "if women intermittent fast, their hormones will be out of whack." This isn't the case, as we will discuss how intermittent fasting truly affects women's hormone as when compared to men.

To briefly talk about men, they were created to "hunt and gather" so to speak. Unlike women, they do not have to carry a baby, which is one of the reasons why intermittent fasting does not affect men as drastically as women. Women are more susceptive to hormones that are related to hunger, and the reason behind is women's reproductive system, as previously mentioned.

The good news is, it will not affect your thyroid as some "experts" will claim, women recognize hunger at a higher degree than men. We recently talked about the Hypothalamus gonadotropin-releasing hormone (GnRH), luteinizing hormone (LH), and follicle-stimulating hormone (FSH), which is responsible for making testosterone and sperm in men and triggering estrogen and ovulation in women.

Women tend to trigger these hormones differently when compared to men, and the main problem occurs because of kisspeptin. For readers that don't know what kisspeptin is, it is a protein-like molecule that neurons use to communicate with each other. Women tend to produce more kisspeptin when compared to men, which is a precursor to (GnRH).

As you know (GnRH) is going to dictate how women produce estrogen and how men are going to produce testosterone; another thing is that kisspeptin is very sensitive to the hunger hormone. If you remember, we mentioned that women are more vulnerable to the hunger hormone when compared to men? The reason behind this is kisspeptin, which causes women to produce less kisspeptin and leads to lower progesterone. In one study done on rats showed that when female rats fast for one day, which is more like a week for women, it caused them to lose 19% of their body weight, but their ovaries shrunk significantly.

Also, they noticed that female rats luteinizing hormone plummeted, and their estrogen levels went through the roof. To briefly touch upon thyroid, t3 levels were deceased. But, t3 levels are always decreasing between meals. The t4, which is responsible for producing thyroid, remained the same, which means the thyroid isn't being affected drastically. It is always suggested that you get regular blood work done to ensure your thyroid is fine, but one of them to tell if it isn't is by seeing how cold you get.

If you feel cold all the time, then the chances are your thyroid is lower. If you notice that you are getting starving throughout the day, and it becomes tough to fast, then break the fast and try it again later. As a woman, you need to listen to your more than men, as women tend to be more sensitive to hormones when intermittent fasting.

Eating enough calories

Since you now know the science behind intermittent fasting and how it can affect women's hormones, let us talk about eating enough calories, especially for women. Believe it or not, this is an important topic to discuss. Especially for women who are much more sensitive to hunger hormones or hormones in general when compared to men. Even though you might be fasting for weight loss, it is critical that you enough calories support your bodily function as a woman. Ideally speaking, women who are trying to lose weight should not eat bellow 200 calories of their maintenance, calculating your maintenance calories the formula is (bodyweight x 12).

Meaning, if your maintenance calories are 2,000 and you are looking to lose weight, then you should not cut it down less than 1,800. If you are someone looking to lose weight with intermittent fasting, we recommend having a macronutrient break down of 20% carbs 50% protein and 30% fats; this shows the percentage of calories coming from specific macronutrients.

We are keeping the carbs low to prevent insulin spikes in check if you are looking to lose weight, we want to keep the insulin as flatlined as possible. However, if you are someone looking to maintain weight and reap the health benefits of intermittent fasting, then we recommend having a macronutrient breakdown of 30% carbs 40% protein 30% fats since we have covered the calorie intake, lets briefly talk about the types of food you should be eating. What you eat to break your fast is just as essential as the number of calories you should be consuming. One thing you need to understand is not to go overboard on the fasting.

As you know, carbs tend to spike your insulin, and when you're fasting, your insulin levels are low, meaning whatever you eat, your body will be sensitive to it. Having spikes of insulin slows down fat loss. Therefore, lower insulin equals more fat burning. If you break your fast with higher amounts of carbs, you will be shutting down the fat burning process. Instead, what we recommend is eating two meals when you break into your eating window. The first one should be lower in carbs and higher in fats and protein; this will ensure you don't turn off your fat burning and get the most out of your fast. The second meal could be higher carbs, and this will help you get ready for the next day if you are fasting.

Another to remember is that your gut will be susceptible to high acidic foods such and drinks, so make sure you stick to foods that are less acidic when you break your fast. Greek yogurt, chicken with some veggies, or even soup works great to break your fast. Now whether your goal is to lose weight or live a healthier life, it is essential that you follow the right calorie intake and macronutrient intake. These tips will go a long way with both the criteria listed.

How to avoid feeling underfed

Since you now know how much to eat, let's talk about how to prevent feeling underfed. Believe it or not, both men and women notice this problem, which causes them to overeat. We need to make sure you don't feed underfed to avoid things like breaking a fast too soon or overeating. There is a couple of technique we can provide you with that shall help you with the feeling of underfed.

The first technique we recommend would be eating wholesome, healthy foods that have a lot of fiber in them. Even though you are free to eat whatever you want, it is still not recommended that you eat unhealthily. When you break your fast, the food you should be eating is high fiber, lower carbs, and moderate protein. What the fiber will do is help you feel fuller throughout the day, making you feel less underfed.

An example of this would be to eat more green leafy vegetables, as they will make you feel fuller for a long time. Since we are on the topic of plants, let us talk about vitamins, you need to have micronutrients dense meals when you are fasting. If you are feeling underfed when fasting, the chances are that you are not consuming enough vitamins and minerals, making you feel underfed.

Make sure you are getting your daily mineral intake during your eating window to avoid such adverse effects; you could take a vitamin supplement during your fasting window to obtain your minerals. But don't use the supplement to take care of your vitamin needs, make sure you are eating healthy foods instead of junk food to feel thoroughly fed. Also, drinking water for the whole day is essential. If you are not drinking enough water, then you have a much higher chance of feeling underfed.

Not only will the water help you feel fuller, but it will also help you to get rid of toxins in your body. Water is a must for a better fasting experience; another thing which can curb your hunger is coffee. If you drink black coffee during your fast, it will help you control any hunger cravings you might be having, which will make you feel less underfed.

One recommendation would be drinking your coffee during the earlier times of the day, instead of later. As drinking coffee then makes you crash pretty hard, which will make you crave more, so make sure you stay away from coffee later during the day. Perhaps consume your coffee earlier in the morning or before your workout works the best, but the main take away would be not to consume junk. Even though fasting allows you to eat whatever you want, it doesn't mean you should, as it can lead you feeling underfed and hungry in the long run. Make sure you are following all these steps to ensure not handling underfed, and as you know, women tend to experience more hunger.

How often should women follow intermittent fasting

When it comes to fasting, women are more sensitive than men. Hence, making the timings and the duration of fasting a bit more restricted than men. Experts suggest that women should have a more relaxed approach than men. This may include shorter fasting days, lesser fasting days, and sometimes eating some food during the fast. We always recommend women to not fast longer than 24 hours, that's why all the fasting protocols listed in this book have a fasting window of no more than 24 hours.

Also, whichever fasting protocol you decide to choose, make sure it is sustainable to you. As it can lead to fewer results overall and disappointment, these being the surface level issues. If women fast for longer than 24 hours, it can lead to hormones going out of whack, and you what could happen then. Another thing to make sure of would be to fast consecutive days in the beginning, and it is recommended that women fast three times a week on consecutive days to ensure they can handle it.

Follow this protocol for the first three weeks, and eventually, if your physician gives you the go, then start lasting longer. With that being said, some women should not follow intermittent fasting. If you are pregnant, trying to conceive, nursing, or under chronic stress, then fasting should not be done. This now brings me to the period women should fast for. Ideally, women should follow a fasting protocol for no longer than eight weeks.

It is ideal for women to take a break from internment fasting after fasting for eight weeks, women should take a whole week off from fasting ideally two weeks off. If you start to notice symptoms such as irregular periods, metabolic stress, anxiety, depression, and insomnia, then stop fasting right away and speak with your doctor. These could be a sign of fasting for too long, so make sure you are looking out for these symptoms every time. There are some fasts you should not do for a prolonged period, such as the 5:2 method and the alternate-day fasting.

For these two fasting protocols, make sure you are not exceeding the six-week mark of following it. Finally, women need to stay on alert when they are fasting, know your body, and make sure you feel right and healthy when you are fasting. Some hunger cravings are fine, but if you start to notice insanity high food cravings which you can't control no matter what, then it is safer to eat some food rather than put your hormones and body in danger.

Fasting can be very fragile in terms of improving health or deteriorating it, especially in women. Which means you need to make sure you ease into fasting and to take regular breaks from it. The timelines we recommend in this chapter works for most women, but consult with a professional before you start or stop a fasting protocol! Good luck.

Symptoms you should look out for

There are many signs to look for when intermittent fasting since you know most of the things related to intermittent fasting by now, let's talk about the significant symptoms to look for. The first one being hunger, many followers of intermittent fasting will notice insane amounts of desire when following intermittent fasting. Which is a given, since you will be going from eating four to six meals throughout the day to none.

The first couple of days will require a ton of willpower to get thru, but eventually, it will subside and get better in a week. Give it some time for your body to get used to intermittent fasting, and be aware of the fact that it will be a shock in the beginning. Besides hunger, cravings for food are very evident when following intermittent fasting. Chances of you breaking your fast will be very high, especially when you are just getting started with it. You will crave foods like a candy bar, fruits, soda's anything which will give you a ton of sugar quickly. You will have to fight these cravings as they will kick in, so make sure you don't indulge in them. Headaches are another thing which beginners might notice.

When you start your intermittent fasting, you will see symptoms such as headaches, don't get worried as they will subside in a week in most cases. Make sure you are drinking plenty of water during your fasting window and after, as this will make it easy for your body to cope with the headaches.

One of the main symptoms you should be looking out for would be feeling cold. You will be contacting cold for the first week, but if it continues past the three-week mark, then consider modifying your fasting protocol. Intermittent fasting has shown to increase blood flow to your fat stores for your body to use it for energy, but if you start feeling cold shivering past the three-week mark, then it is a symptom you should be looking out.

Since you will be drinking a lot of water, this will make you feel even colder throughout the day, so unless you feel cold, don't take it seriously. Speaking of drinking water, you will also notice you going to the bathroom a lot. It is because of your water consumption, and there isn't a way around it since we don't recommend you drink less water. These are the main symptoms you will notice when you first start intermittent fasting, and they usually last three weeks.

If you experience these symptoms at the same magnitude as you were the first week, then please modify your fasting protocol as it might not be suitable for your body. If you healthily want to follow intermittent fasting, then it is best to look out for these symptoms and to listen to your body. If you're going to avoid these symptoms, then ease into intermittent fasting and making sure it isn't a shock for your body from the get-go.

Tips for intermittent fasting for women

Let's talk about some quick tips women need to consider before they start intermittent fasting, as there are some great ones to find before you start. The first tip would be to drink a ton of water when fasting, pretty easy to follow and understand. You need to drink water to curb your cravings, as you know, women tend to crave foods more than men do only because of the hormone response.

Drinking water will also help you control the headache symptoms you might get; overall, drinking water is a must. Drinking tea and coffee will help you manage your hunger throughout the day; it will also give you more energy in the beginning stages of fasting.

Just make sure you drink black coffee or black/green tea, don't add any sugar or milk as it will break your fast if you do that. If you find yourself around people who aren't supportive of your fasting endeavors, then make sure you stay away from them or at least avoid talking about fasting. The last thing you want is unsupportive people when you are following intermittent fasting, so make sure you stay away from them and stay positive. Finally, give yourself at least a month when you start intermittent fasting.

Many people don't realize that it will take some time to start seeing changes in their body; four weeks is a good time for your body to begin adapting to intermittent fasting. Meaning, you need to keep up the fast for at least a month for you to make a judgment whether fasting is for you or not, and most of the time, it works out in your favor. In the first four weeks of fasting, you will notice hunger waves avoid them by drinking coffee or tea. The main tip when intermittent fasting would be to not binge eat when you break your fast, you will have the craving to binge eat.

Avoid it. Follow our macros and eating patterns, which we have listed above in this. If you want to develop your eating pattern, that's fine as well; make sure not a lot of carbs are on your plate in your first meal as this will make you binge eat later. Making sure you don't overeat is essential for intermittent fasting, as it will dictate your goals. If you are looking to lose weight, then make sure you eat portion-controlled meals instead of eating whatever your heart desires. These are all the primary tips, make sure you follow them, so you don't end up giving up too soon.

All in all, these tips will help you in the future. As you will see, how much easier fasting becomes for you once you start considering these tips, but don't forget to listen to your body as we previously mentioned. Looking out for your health first is very important, so if you feel like these tips are not helping you within three weeks, then modify your fasting.

Chapter 7: Manage the Symptoms of Menopause

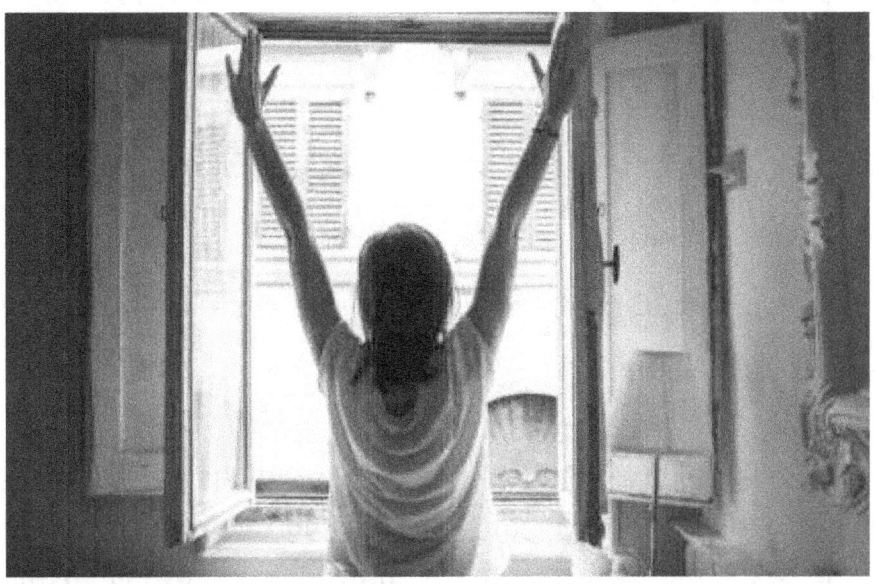

We will discuss all of the issues someone might face when following intermittent fasting, we will also touch upon menopause and how to take care of it appropriately. Intermittent fasting truly is a great way to live the life you want. We will give you all the good and the bad about intermittent fasting, getting you all geared up to get started.

Don't Test the Limits

You must never try to stretch the fasting too far. You have to fast and then give your body the time to recover. If you are beginning fasting, never fast on consecutive days. Always allow your body the time to recover.

Don't Fast Too Long

Initially, you should begin by creating safe gaps between your meals. Eliminate snacks. Then try to stretch the difference between the meals a bit. Always ensure that the highest amount of time spent without food is at the beginning of the fast. It means it is still better to begin fasts early in the evening as you will not feel hungry. Stretching your fast for too long in the morning wouldn't be a very bright idea. In any case, the fasting duration should be anywhere between 12-14 hours only. Several studies have shown that women get much better results with comparatively shorter fasts than men.

No HIIT on Fasting Days

High-intensity interval training is an energy-demanding activity. It should be avoided at all costs on the fasting days, especially if you are beginning your intermittent fasting. It can drain you and create intense energy demands.

No Fasting During the Menstrual Cycle

There is significant blood loss during the periods, and your body needs a lot of rest. Your hormones are also going crazy during this time. Therefore, you must not practice intermittent fasting at this time. Have a Healthy Diet Food choices are critical in the case of women as their nutritional requirements are high.

You must choose a very healthy diet full of all the nutrients so that your hormones remain in check. You should stop fasting if you notice the following things:

- Irregular periods or complete absence of periods

- Sudden resurfacing of sleep disorders without any apparent reason

- On facing sudden and drastic metabolic and digestive issues

- On experiencing sudden mood swings and brain fog

- On having sudden changes in the color of the skin or hair texture

Intermittent Fasting is NOT for you if:

- You have eating disorders

- Have got pregnant or trying to conceive

- Have sleep disorders

- Have adrenal fatigue

- You are suffering from PMS, PCOS, PCOD, Fibroids, Endometriosis, or other hormonal issues

Intermittent fasting isn't a diet. It is a routine. Diets are restrictive; routines are liberating as they flow with life. You always find time to do things while following a method as they are just a part of life. I don't believe people on diets would be able to say the same.

So, you must make it clear in your mind that intermittent fasting isn't a diet. The biggest reason for foods to fail is that they put so many restrictions that people may or may not lose their weight, but they lose their peace of mind. Imagine yourself at a party with people eating and merrymaking. Then imagine yourself standing in one corner sulking as you can't eat anything. Most of the food items that you like are there, but you can't have them.

The steel-clad resolve of sticking to the diet flies out of the window that very moment. The people who can keep the resolve start developing a feeling of resentment. Food is an essential requirement in life. It is needed for satisfying physical, mental, and emotional needs. Anything that is so restrictive cannot be adopted as a lifestyle. Intermittent fasting, on the other hand, is very simple. You only need to remain in the fasted state for a set number of hours in a day or a week.

The kind of diet you want to have, the amount of food you want to eat and the number of hours you want to spend doing an exercise can be up to your own choice. These will all help you in losing weight and staying healthier; however, you would still lose weight even if you don't eat the prescribed food items or don't sweat in the gym for long.

The most significant advantage of intermittent fasting is that it can be quickly adopted as a lifestyle. You don't need to do anything out of the ordinary to follow intermittent fasting. You don't need to prepare elaborate meals. You don't need to be choosy every time you have to decide to eat something. Healthy eating is always advisable, but that doesn't mean you have to get extra picky. Intermittent fasting is a straightforward routine where you will have a certain number of hours in a day to eat. The remaining hours will be the fasting hours, and in them, you can't have anything besides the exempted items listed on the meal plan.

The best thing is that after some time of practicing intermittent fasting, staying hungry for extra-long wouldn't remain a problem at all. It is more about when to eat and less about what or how much to eat Intermittent fasting lays great emphasis on when to eat.

The simple reasons for that are:

• Frequent meals cause significant damage to our system as they keep our gut under constant pressure.

• The blood sugar levels remain consistently high as you keep eating food at short intervals.

• The insulin spike is also there, and hence, you remain prone to insulin sensitivity.

• It also increases cholesterol levels.

• Chronic inflammation also rises.

• Your body is not able to achieve satiety.

• Organs need to work extra hard to adjust the extra energy. All this can be avoided by simply reducing the number of meals in a day. You don't need to reduce the number of calories you have in a day.

You can still have your 2000 calories if you like. You can have even more if you want. You can also eat the pancakes once in a while and again lose weight because your body now has the time to focus on other things besides just digesting food. The human body has passed through a long evolutionary process, and hence, it knows the methods that can help it run smoothly. The recent overexposure to food has complicated things a bit as the body not only gets busy in dealing with the extra energy, but it also has to deal with food items that are not very healthy. Once you start giving it the time to digest the food and begin the necessary processes, it can quickly deal with the kind of food you eat.

Therefore, the real emphasis in intermittent fasting would always remain on maintaining the fasting state for a definite period in a day. We can divide the day into two segments:

The Fasting Window: This is the time of the day during which you can't eat anything at all. There are some exceptions like unsweetened black tea or coffee, unsweetened fresh lime water, or green tea that you can still have in this period as these don't add any calories or don't initiate your digestive process. Besides these items in limited quantity, you need to remain in a completely fasted state during this period. The fasting window is comparatively more prolonged than the eating window.

However, you can set the duration of the fasting window as per your convenience and tolerance.

The Eating Window: This is the time of the day during which you can eat. It is always advisable to have a smaller number of meals in a day. You must try to eliminate snacks and unnecessary munching as it leads to cravings and also causes insulin resistance, however, you can eat your fill in your eating windows. There are no calorie caps in intermittent fasting protocols. You need to make your meals as fulfilling as possible so that you don't feel the need to have snacks in between your meals. Healthy food items in the meals are always excellent. They would help you in fighting obesity and chronic inflammation.

However, you can bring these changes one at a time, and there will not be a need to rush the process. The most important part of this to remember will always be to maintain fasting and eating windows.

Things to make everything easy for you.

Exercise and especially, high-intensity interval training, works wonders if you are following intermittent fasting. The reason is simple; intermittent fasting boosts the production of hormones that can increase fat burn. High-intensity interval training creates the right environment at the right time. You may be engaging in high-intensity physical activity later in the day too. But the effects wouldn't be the same as at that time; you would be in a fed state. In that case, there will be no presence of HGH in your bloodstream. This is a hormone which can only be present when you are on an empty stomach after a long fasting interval. It acts as a potent steroid, which is so potent that sports organizations have banned its use as it improves the performance of the athletes.

Therefore, exercise works in intermittent fasting. Not only high-intensity interval training but light cardio exercises, yoga, and aerobics also have their definitive health benefits. If you want to reap the full benefits of intermittent fasting, you must include training in your schedule.

Healthy Food

In this whole book, we have stressed the least on food. It has been intentional so that you can focus entirely on the process and its advantages. However, this doesn't mean that food doesn't play an essential role in fulfilling your objectives, or it isn't crucial. First, healthy food is necessary.

You must try to consume as much fresh and unprocessed food as possible. Staying away from syrups, juices, jam, and jellies is always advisable as these things increase the number of calories consumed but don't give anything to your body. You must always avoid such situations. Still, eat fruits with their pulp. Throwing away the flesh and drinking only the juice is the most significant loss you will face ever. Maintaining a balance among the macronutrients is also very important as reducing the number of meals consumed in a day also affects your calorie intake. If you do not have a balanced diet, you can get nutrient deficient. Therefore, having a healthy diet helps in burning body fat and reducing weight. If your goal is explicitly fat burning, then you should take a keto diet along with intermittent fasting. Keto diet is a high-fat, low-carb diet that helps your body in switching to burning solid fuel in place of glucose fuel. Once that process begins, fat burning becomes very fast and effective. This is simply a suggestion, and you can make do with any healthy eating plan. Recipes will be available for you in this book.

A Positive Attitude

Your attitude plays a vital role whenever bringing any change is considered. With a pessimistic attitude, a person may even lose hope of success or survival is falling even in a small pool. It is not the swimming skills that keep a person afloat but the will and confidence to survive. Recently, a Mexican survived in the Pacific Ocean for 438 days. No amount of swimming skills could have saved a person for that long in the Pacific. However, it was the optimism and will to survive that kept him alive. Weight loss can get disappointing and disheartening at times.

The reaction of people and over conscious attitude at times makes people look for faster results, and they don't follow procedure and then fail. Such things should never be taken to heart. You must always have confidence and the will to succeed. You must keep making adjustments to get the desired results, but looking for shortcuts can lead to failures. Health should always be a long-term goal, as this is the only thing that matters in the end.

Chapter 8: Recipes + 10-Day Plan

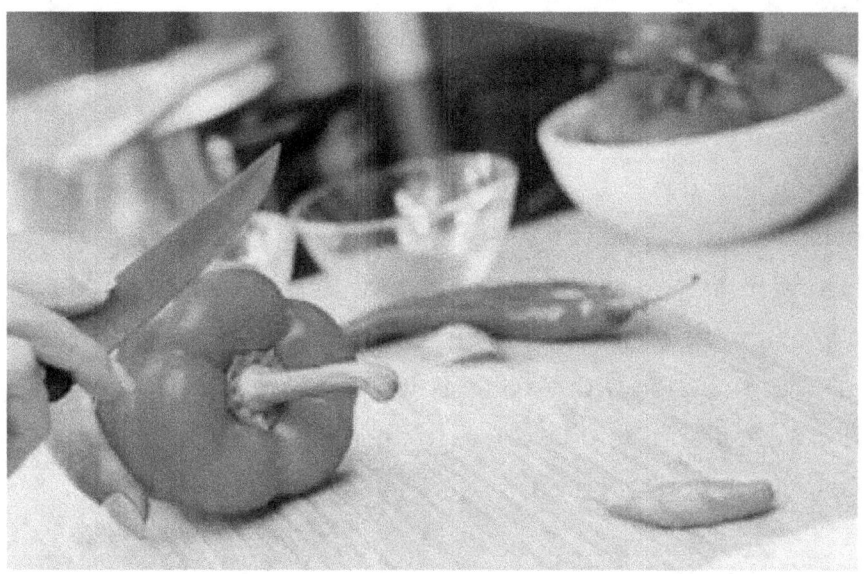

In this chapter, we will be giving you some fantastic low calories recipes, which will not only help you to lose body fat and to put on muscle. These recipes are very low in calories, which will allow you to fill up quite quickly, and they're also nutritionally dense that will also allow you to be more successful in putting on muscle losing fat or whatever it is that you're trying to achieve. The great thing about intermittent fasting is that it is ideal for any goal; the main benefits of intermittent fasting is to detoxify you and to be overall healthy being.

10-Day Plan

Now in this chapter, we will also help you to figure out the right eating plan and give you a 10-day for eating plans that you are in a high position to not only put on muscle or to lose fat butt to make intermittent fasting a habit. This is the main take away from this book, you need to make sure that you make intermittent fasting your practices of a you start seeing the results that you have been looking for Now we will a general example of how you will be eating in a 16/8 fasting protocol, as making a full eating plan could be redundant and pointless, as it is very easy to make the eating plan yourself once you get the idea behind it.

That being said, let's give you the eating plan. This plan is based on your fasting from 6:30 am till 10 am, I know this isn't exactly 16 hours, but half an hour here and there is fine. This protocol will work great for you, in conjunction with the fantastic recipes we have to offer you. The trick with intermittent fasting is to find tasty foods to eat during your fast, so you don't regret it.

Meal 1: 10- 10:30

Breakfast recipes from below

Meal 2: 12 - 12:30

Snack

Meal 3: 3 - 3:30

Lunch recipe from below

Meal 4: 6 - 6:30

Dinner recipes from below

Follow this eating plan for ten days, and you should be in a high position to seeing amazing results and to make this a full-blown habit. The main take away would be to make intermittent fasting an eating habit instead of a diet.

Breakfast

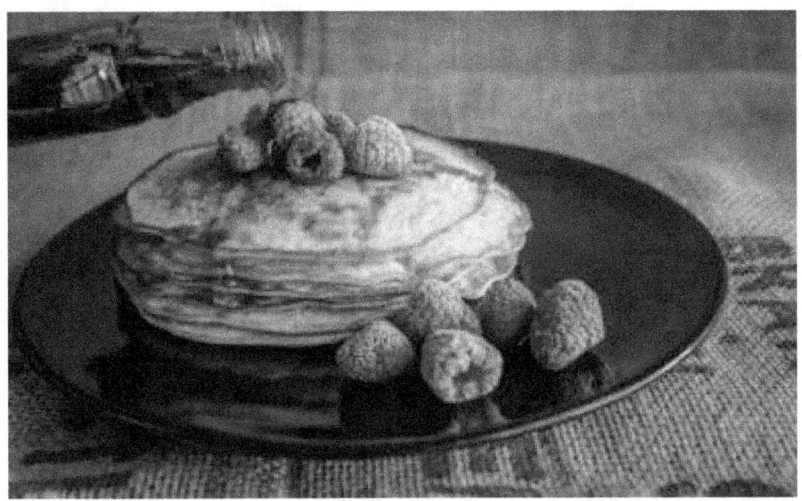

Crustless Broccoli Sun-dried Tomato Quiche

This crustless tofu quiche is low in cholesterol and high in protein. This can be served hot or cold and can be made in muffin tins for an on-the-go breakfast that packs a protein punch.

Ingredients:

12.3-ounce box extra-firm tofu drained and dried

1 ½ cup broccoli, chopped

2 leeks, cleaned and sliced; both white and green parts

2 tablespoons vegetable broth

3 tablespoons nutritional yeast

2 chopped cloves of garlic

1 lemon, juiced

2 teaspoons yellow mustard

1 tablespoon tahini

1 tablespoon cornstarch

¼ cup old fashioned oats

½ teaspoon turmeric

3-4 dashes Tabasco sauce

½-1 teaspoon salt

½ cup artichoke hearts, chopped

2/3 cup tomatoes, sun-dried, soaked in hot water

1/8 cup vegetable broth

Instructions:

- Preheat your oven to 375 degrees Fahrenheit.
- Prepare a 9" pie plate or springform pan with parchment paper or cooking spray.
- Put all of the leeks and broccoli on a cookie sheet and drizzle with vegetable broth, salt, and pepper. Bake for about 20-30 min.

- In the meantime, add the tofu, garlic, nutritional yeast, lemon juice, mustard, tahini, cornstarch, oats, turmeric, salt, and a few dashes of Tabasco in a food processor. When the mixture is smooth, taste for heat and add more Tabasco as needed.

- Place cooked vegetables with artichoke hearts and tomatoes in a large bowl. With a spatula, scrape in tofu mixture from the processor. Mix carefully, so all of the vegetables are well distributed. If the mixture seems too dry, add a little vegetable broth or water.

- Add mixture to pie plate muffin tins, or springform pan and spread evenly.

- Bake for about 35 min. or until lightly browned.

- Cool before serving. It is delicious, both warm and chilled!

Chocolate Pancakes

Everyone deserves chocolate for breakfast every once in a while. Satisfy your sweet tooth with these gluten-free, vegan chocolate pancakes that go well with almost any fruit of choice, especially strawberries, bananas, and raspberries.

Ingredients:

1 ¼ cup gluten-free flour of choice

1 tablespoon ground flaxseed

1 tablespoon baking powder

3 tablespoons nutritional yeast

2 tablespoons unsweetened cocoa powder

¼ teaspoon of sea salt

1 cup unsweetened, unflavored almond milk

1 tablespoon vegan mini chocolate chips (optional)

1 teaspoon vanilla extract

¼ teaspoon stevia powder or 1 tablespoon pure maple syrup

1 tablespoon apple cider vinegar

¼ cup unsweetened applesauce.

Instructions:

- Get a medium bowl and mix all the dry ingredients (flour, baking powder, flaxseed, cocoa powder, yeast, salt, and optional chocolate chips). Whisk until evenly combined.

- In a separate small bowl, combine wet ingredients except for the applesauce (almond milk, vanilla extract, apple cider vinegar, maple syrup, or stevia powder).

- Add wet ingredient mixture and applesauce to the dry ingredients and mix by hand until ingredients are just combined.

- The batter should sit for 10 minutes. It will rise and thicken, possibly doubling in size.

- Heat an electric griddle or nonstick skillet to medium heat and spray with a small amount of nonstick spray, if desired. Scoop batter into 3-inch rounds. Much like traditional pancakes, bubbles will start to appear. When bubbles start to burst, flip pancakes and cook for 1-2 minutes. Yields 12 pancakes.

Breakfast Scramble

Here is another egg-free breakfast option for the veggie lover! Many scramble recipes call for tofu, whereas here we are using cauliflower. This recipe is versatile and allows you to use whichever veggies you may already have in your refrigerator. Feel free to substitute at will!

Ingredients:

1 large head cauliflower, cut up

1 seeded, diced green bell pepper

1 seeded, diced red bell pepper

2 cups sliced mushrooms (approximately 8 oz whole mushrooms)

1 peeled, diced red onion

3 peeled, minced cloves of garlic

Sea salt

1 ½ teaspoons turmeric

1–2 tablespoons of low-sodium soy sauce

¼ cup nutritional yeast (optional)

½ teaspoon black pepper

Instructions:

1. Sauté green and red peppers, mushrooms, and onion in a medium saucepan or skillet over medium-high heat until onion is translucent (should be 7–8 min). Add an occasional tablespoon or two of water to the pan to prevent vegetables from sticking.

2. Add cauliflower and cook until florets are tenders. It should be 5 to 6 minutes.

3. Add, pepper, garlic, soy sauce, turmeric, and yeast (if using) to the pan and cook for about 5 minutes.

Superfood Breakfast Bars

Need a quick pre-made breakfast option you can grab and go? This breakfast bar is not only sweet and salty, but it's also vegan, gluten-free, and packed with superfood energy.

Ingredients:

4 apples

1.5 cups mix of mulberries and goji berries, soaked in lukewarm water for about 30 minutes

1 cup all-natural apple juice + 3 tablespoons divided

2 tablespoons maple syrup

2-3 tablespoons sunflower seed butter

2 teaspoons aluminum-free baking powder

4 cups gluten-free certified oats

Pinch of cinnamon (optional)

Sunflower seeds for garnish

Instructions:

1. Preheat your oven to 390 degrees Fahrenheit.

2. Line the 11" x 8" baking dish with parchment paper.

3. Chop apples coarsely and remove seeds. Add to blender with 1 c. of the apple juice. Blend until smooth

4. Mix the remaining 3 tablespoons of apple juice, sunflower butter, and maple syrup in a small bowl. You will create a creamy and smooth paste.

5. In a large bowl, combine the soaked and trained berries, oats, sunflower paste, baking powder, and apple mix into a well-mixed dough.

6. Press the dough with a spatula or your hands in the baking dish. Top it with sunflower seeds. Bake for 20 min.

Lunch

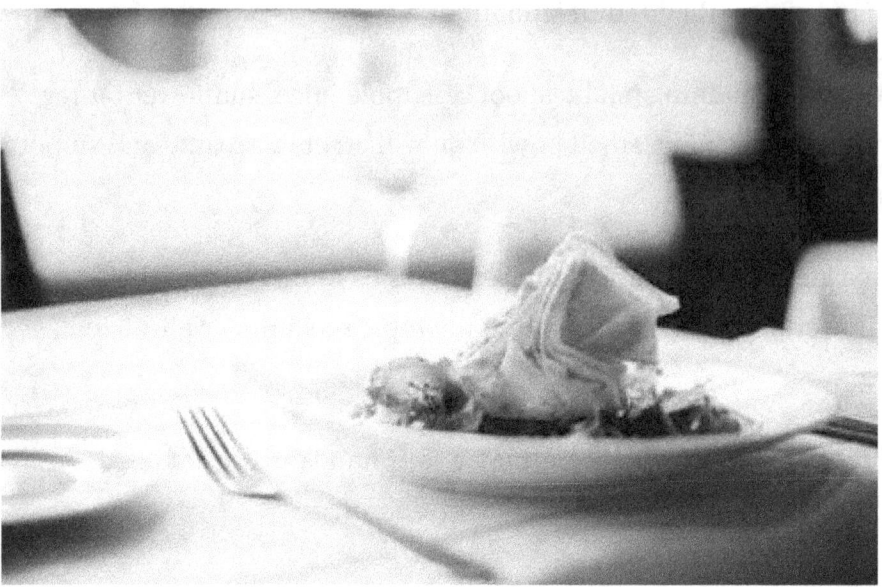

Vegan Tuna Salad

This "tuna salad" recipe includes inexpensive, easy to find ingredients that can be made in advance and stored in the refrigerator for about a week. Serve on a bed of greens, your favorite crackers, or as a classic sandwich. Feel free to add ingredients for flavor and texture, such as carrots or bell peppers.

Ingredients:

2 cans chickpeas

1 tablespoon prepared yellow mustard

2 tablespoons vegan mayonnaise

1 tablespoon jarred capers

2 tablespoons pickle relish

½ cup chopped celery

Instructions:

1. In a medium bowl, combine chickpeas, mustard, vegan mayo, and mustard. Pulse in a food processor or mash with a potato masher until the mixture is partially smooth with some chunks.

2. Add the remaining ingredients to the chickpea mixture and mix until combined.

3. Serve immediately or refrigerate until ready to serve.

Veggie Wrap with Apples and Spicy Hummus

Wraps are a versatile and portable lunch option that can be adapted to any taste. The combination of the soft hummus and broccoli slaw creates a balanced texture of smoothness and crunchiness. The spicy hummus with apple brings a unique sweet and spicy blend. The end result: a lunch wrap that is anything but boring.

Ingredients:

1 tortilla of your choice: flour, corn, gluten-free, etc.

3-4 tablespoons of your favorite spicy hummus (a plain hummus mixed with salsa is good, too!)

A few leaves of your favorite leafy greens

¼ apple sliced thin

½ cup broccoli slaw (store-bought or homemade are both good)

½ teaspoon lemon juice

2 teaspoons dairy-free, plain, unsweetened yogurt

Salt and pepper to taste

Instructions:

1. Mix broccoli slaw with lemon juice and yogurt. Add pepper and salt to taste and mix well.

2. Lay tortilla flat.

3. Spread hummus all over the tortilla.

4. Lay down leafy greens on hummus.

5. On one half, pile broccoli slaw over lettuce. Place apples on top of the slaw.

6. Starting with the half with slaw and apples, roll tortilla tightly.

7. Cut in half if desired and enjoy!

Mac and Cheese Bites

Welcome to the vegan twist on an old classic. We promised this book would help satisfy some of your old, pre-vegan cravings, so here's a great portable comfort food bite that will satisfy kids and grown-ups alike. Note that these can be eaten warm or cool, though warming them up may make them fall apart a bit.

Ingredients:

1 ½ cups uncooked macaroni (gluten-free will work if needed)

1 medium onion, chopped (can substitute with 1 medium yellow pepper if you don't care for onions.)

1 clove garlic, chopped

2 tablespoons cornstarch, or arrowroot powder

1 cup non-dairy milk

½ teaspoon smoked paprika (can substitute for chipotle powder)

1 teaspoon lemon juice or apple cider vinegar

½ cup nutritional yeast

1 teaspoon salt

Instructions:

1. Preheat your oven to 350 degrees Fahrenheit.

2. Prepare the muffin tin with liners.

3. Prepare macaroni according to instructions.

4. While macaroni is cooking, sauté garlic and onion (or substitute of choice) until it is just starting to turn golden brown. This can be done in a dry pan, but adding some oil will work as well.

5. Add garlic, onion, and all other non-macaroni ingredients into a blender and mix until smooth.

6. Drain the macaroni and return to the pan.

7. Pour sauce over macaroni and stir well.

8. Spoon mixture into muffin tin, stirring occasionally in between such an equal amount of sauce goes in each cup.

9. Push down tops with the back of a spoon.

10. Bake in the oven for 30 min.

11. Serve once cooled.

Chick'n Salad with Cranberries and Pistachios

This recipe calls for soy curls (or textured vegetable protein) for the "chick'n," but you could easily use tempeh or another meat substitute for choice. This salad can be served on a bed of greens, put into a wrap, or on bread as a traditional sandwich.

Ingredients:

1 ½ cups dry soy curls (textured vegetable protein)

2 dashes apple cider vinegar

½ cup diced granny smith apples (approx. 1 small apple)

¼ cup shelled pistachios, chopped

½ cup dried cranberries

5-6 tablespoons veganaise (adjust depending on how creamy you would like the salad to be)

1 teaspoon of sea salt

A pinch of thyme

Instructions:

1. Soak soy curls in warm water for 10 min. Squeeze excess water out of them and roughly chop larger pieces. Set aside.

2. While soy curls are soaking, mix diced apple and vinegar. Drain any excess liquid.

3. Combine apples with all other ingredients in large bowl until ingredients are evenly mixed. Add seasoning to taste. Chill for at least 30 minutes. Serve as desired.

Dinner

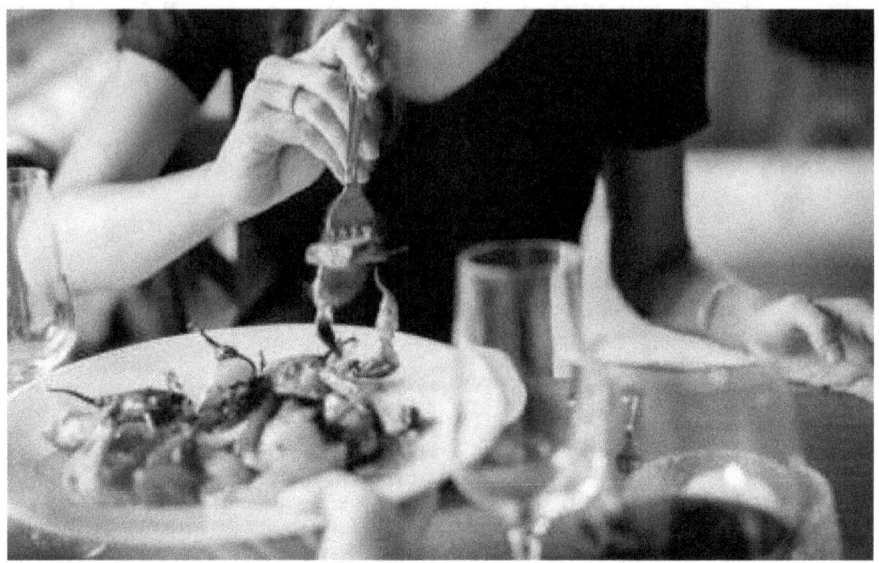

End the day with these satisfying, belly-filling dinners that are great for families and solo homes alike.

Pan-fried Jackfruit over Pasta with Lemon Coconut Cream Sauce

This creamy, lemony coconut sauce can be served with a variety of meat alternatives. Jackfruit gives the dish a hint of sweetness to break through the richness of the cream sauce.

Ingredients:

1 lb. pasta of choice

2 cans jackfruit in brine

2 tablespoons flour of choice

Garlic powder, dried oregano, paprika, black pepper, kosher salt to taste

2 tablespoons vegetable oil

4 tablespoons vegan butter

2 cups of coconut milk

Juice of 1 lemon

2 tablespoons grated vegan parmesan cheese

1 pinch ground nutmeg

1 teaspoon lemon zest (can use the same lemon from juice)

Fresh basil leaves, chopped for garnish

Instructions:

1. Cook pasta until al dente. Drain the pasta but reserve 1 cup of the pasta water. Set it aside for now.

2. While the pasta is cooking, drain the jackfruit and cut each piece in half. Pat jackfruit dry.

3. Mix flour with garlic powder, oregano, paprika, pepper, and salt in a separate bowl.

4. Toss flour mixture with jackfruit.

5. Heat vegetable oil in a skillet. Pan-fry the jackfruit until crisp on both sides. It takes around ten minutes in total.

6. Transfer the jackfruit to a plate lined with a paper towel and set aside.

7. In a large saucepan or skillet, melt vegan butter. Add coconut milk and lemon juice. Then add parmesan cheese and nutmeg. Cook until sauce is thick.

8. Add cooked pasta and half of the reserved pasta water to skillet. Toss to coat all pasta.

9. Cook until everything is hot and the sauce is to desired consistency and pasta is heated through. If the sauce is too thick, continue to use remaining pasta water.

10. Turn off heat. Add lemon zest and add pepper and salt to taste. Sprinkle parmesan and basil leaves. Add pan-fried jackfruit on top when serving.

Butternut Squash Tacos with Tempeh Chorizo

This dish comes together quite easily, though there are a few preparation tips recommended you do in advance. If you have challenges with digesting beans or soy, steam your tempeh before using it. Simmer the butternut squash in veggie broth or water and vinegar as this adds more flavor in lieu of steaming. Keep a little extra water on hand in case the squash starts to stick.

Ingredients:

One 8-ounce package tempeh

½ cup of filtered water

¼ cup apple cider vinegar

2 cups butternut squash, peeled, cut into cubes

1 teaspoon chili powder

½ teaspoon smoked paprika

½ teaspoon cumin

½ teaspoon garlic powder

½ teaspoon oregano

A dash of cayenne

1 tablespoon nutritional yeast

A few dashes of liquid smoke

Black pepper and sea salt to taste

½ cup thinly julienned carrot (optional)

8 corn tortillas (or whatever you have on hand)

1 large avocado, pitted and sliced

Cilantro, chopped

Instructions:

1. Cut the tempeh into two parts. Steam for 10 min. Place in a large bowl and tear apart into small pieces either with your hands (after it's cooled) or with a pastry cutter.

2. While tempeh is steaming, bring water and vinegar to a boil in a small skillet.

3. Add spices, squash, liquid smoke, nutritional yeast, and a pinch of sea salt to skillet. Coat well and simmer covered, stirring occasionally. Add carrots and tempeh, covering again. Simmer a little while longer, stirring to prevent sticking. Uncover and season with pepper and salt.

4. Fill warmed tortillas with squash and tempeh mix and top with avocado and cilantro.

Vegan Fish Sticks and Tartar Sauce

This recipe for the so-called "wish" sticks as some call it. This has been kid-tested and approved, though adults can enjoy them on a sandwich or a salad topper.

Ingredients:

Fish Sticks:

12-ounce package extra-firm tofu

½ cup cornmeal

1 tablespoon garlic powder

1 tablespoon dried basil

2 tablespoons dulse flakes

1 tablespoon onion powder

½ cup whole wheat flour (rice flour is a good gluten-free option)

10 turns fresh black pepper

1 tablespoon of sea salt

¼ cup non-dairy milk, unsweetened

1 cup high-heat oil for frying

Vegan Tartar Sauce:

¼ cup sweet pickle relish

½ cup vegan mayo

½ teaspoon sugar

½ teaspoon lemon juice

5 turns fresh black pepper

Instructions:

1. Rinse tofu and drain in a colander. Placing a heavy plate on tofu with a heavy item on top will help drain better. Set it aside.

2. In a medium bowl, mix the flour, cornmeal, garlic powder, basil, onion powder, dulse flakes, pepper, and salt. Whisk together. Set the mix aside.

3. Set tofu on cutting board. Cut into quarters.

4. Slice tofu into thin pieces. You should have 28-32 pieces in total.

5. In a large cast-iron skillet, heat oil on medium/low heat.

6. In a small bowl, pour non-dairy milk.

7. Dip each piece of tofu in non-dairy milk. Immediately dip in breading, coating all sides evenly. Repeat until all pieces are coated.

8. The oil will start to splatter when hot enough. At that point, add tofu pieces to skillet. Repeat until all pieces are cooked.

9. Each side will cook for about 2-3 minutes. Watch for golden brown color. Place tofu pieces on a brown paper bag as you remove them from pan to soak up excess oil.

10. Repeat as necessary until all tofu is cooked. Cool before serving. Mix all tartar sauce ingredients until an even and creamy sauce is made. Enjoy!

Vegan Philly Cheesesteak

A great twist on a regional favorite, this sandwich is fairly simple to put together and contains ingredients that are easy to find. It can be served with vegan mayo if desired.

Ingredients:

6-8 sliced Portobello mushrooms

4 cloves garlic, minced

1 tablespoon olive oil

1 whole clove garlic

½ teaspoon black pepper

1 teaspoon dried thyme

½ large diced onion

A dash of kosher salt

1 tablespoon vegan Worcestershire sauce

Hoagie rolls or another small loaf of bread of choice

1 cup shredded vegan cheddar cheese

Vegan mayo (optional)

Instructions:

1. Preheat the broiler.

2. In a deep skillet, heat olive oil. Brown mushrooms in oil, about 10 min.

3. Add thyme, garlic, and pepper until evenly coated.

4. Add onion and salt. Mushrooms must be well cooked before adding salt. Cook until onion is caramelized and softened, which should be for about 5 minutes. Add Worcestershire sauce and mix well.

5. Slice the bread lengthwise. Coat open sides of bread with olive oil or cooking spray. To add garlic flavor, cut the whole garlic clove, cut off the tip, and put on the oiled side of bread. Garlic powder is also a good substitute.

6. If desired, add optional vegan mayo. Place bread on cookie sheet. Fill loaves with mushrooms and top with shredded vegan cheddar cheese.

7. Place in broiler until cheese has melted, which should be 4-5 minutes.

Desserts and Snacks

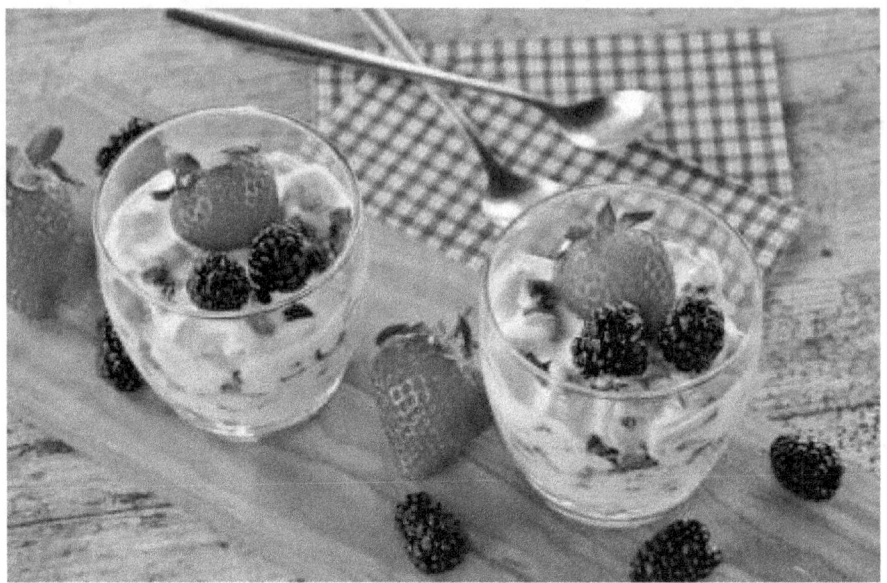

Switching to a refined sugar-free, plant-based lifestyle doesn't have to mean depriving yourself of your sweet tooth cravings. Make these for your own late-night treat or multiply the ingredients for family gatherings.

Mango Lime Chia Pudding

Chia pudding is another versatile treat that can be used at breakfast or as a mid-day snack. Pack it in a mason jar or a recycled food jar. This is one of many flavor combinations you can create.

Ingredients:

3 cups fresh or frozen mango chunks

One 15.5-ounce can coconut milk

1 tablespoon lime zest

¼ cup maple syrup

¼ cup freshly squeezed lime juice

¼ cup hemp seeds

1/3 cup chia seeds

Topping options: Approximately 8 cups of any combination of mango, banana, pineapple, or any fruit you'd love with mango and lime. (Banana is a fruit you'd want to wait to add until you are ready to eat the pudding as it browns and gets mushy very quickly once out of its peel)

Instructions:

1. Place mango chunks, coconut milk, lime zest, and maple syrup in a blender. Mix until smooth.

2. Add hemp and chia seeds in the blender and stir by hand or blend on low to just combine.

3. This should yield 4 cups of pudding. Portion it as you prefer. One suggestion is to divide into 8 portions, one each in a pint jar, and top with one cup of fresh fruit.

4. Refrigerate pudding until ready to eat, minimum 4 hours to set. The pudding keeps for 5-7 days.

Mint Chocolate Truffle Larabar Bites

This copycat recipe can be rolled into individual balls or placed in a pan and cut up as bars after firming in the refrigerator. With 15-minute prep time, this quick fix will satisfy any sweet tooth! Can keep for 3 weeks if refrigerated in an airtight container.

Ingredients:

1 cup vegan chocolate chips (semi-sweet dark chips are recommended)

10 large Medjool dates

1 ½ cups of raw almonds

¼ cup coconut flour

¼ cup of cocoa powder

¼-1/2 teaspoon peppermint extract

2 tablespoons water

Instructions:

1. Pour almonds into a food processor and chop until a fine flour.

2. Add chocolate chips, dates, flour and cocoa, and process again until well combined.

3. Add oil and peppermint extract.

4. Process one more time until the mix starts balling up.

5. Taste a small bit and add more peppermint if you wish. Process again if you do.

6. Remove the blade from the processor and form the dough into balls. Choose whatever size you like, as they do not need to bake and will be good in any portion.

Peanut Butter Caramel Rice Krispies

Take a trip down memory lane and bring the wonderful memory of rice Krispie treats into the adult world. This healthier version will give you a light and crunchy snack that is great for munching at home or family potlucks.

Ingredients:

6 cups crisp rice cereal

1/3 cup creamy peanut butter (can substitute with almond or sunflower seed butter)

¾ cup brown rice syrup

1 teaspoon vanilla extract

¼ cup maple syrup

Peanut butter drizzle:

2 tablespoons creamy peanut butter (or substitute of choice)

1 teaspoon maple syrup (or another liquid sweetener)

1-2 teaspoons to thin, if needed

Instructions:

1. Line a 9" x 9" square pan with parchment or wax paper. An 8" x 8" pan will work as well. Treats will just be thicker.

2. Place a large pot over medium heat. Add brown rice syrup and maple syrup in and bring it to a rolling boil. Cook for 1-2 minutes, stirring often and making sure mix does not burn.

3. Remove from heat. Mix in vanilla and peanut butter with whisk until smooth.

4. In a large bowl, pour in crisp rice cereal. Stir in the liquid mix until well combined.

5. Scoop into pan and spread out evenly. Press down with wet fingers or spatula. Place in freezer to set for 10 minutes while making peanut butter drizzle.

6. In a separate microwavable bowl, mix together peanut butter and maple syrup. Microwave in 30-second intervals until just warm for easier mixing. Add 1 teaspoon water at a time if needed. Mix until smooth.

7. Remove treats from the freezer and drizzle on the peanut butter mix. Place back in the freezer until firm, about 10 min.

8. Cut into squares for serving. Bars will hold their shape quite well at room temperature but can be stored in the fridge. Leftovers can be wrapped up and kept in the fridge for 5 to 7 days or freeze for up to one month.

Easy Chocolate Pudding

Get ready to throw away the instant boxed stuff and try this equally easy, dairy-free chocolate pudding that is so rich, creamy, and chocolatey that you won't believe that it's healthy and refined sugar-free. Top with coconut whipped cream for a perfect treat.

Ingredients:

1 ½ cups organic coconut cream from a can

½ cup raw cacao powder (sifted unsweetened cocoa powder works as well)

6 tablespoons pure maple syrup (may adjust to up to 8 tablespoons, depending on how sweet you like it)

2 teaspoons pure vanilla extract

Fine-grain sea salt

Instructions:

1. In a small saucepan over low heat, whisk coconut cream, cacao, and maple syrup until smooth. A smaller whisk my make a smoother mixture. Continue to cook over low/medium for 2 minutes, or until the mixture just starts to come to a boil with small bubbles.

2. Remove from heat. Add salt and vanilla. Stir. Taste and add more maple if you'd like a sweeter pudding.

3. Pour into individual containers/bowls or keep in one larger bowl to set.

4. Cover and refrigerate until set, or overnight for a thick and creamy pudding. Makes 4 servings.

CONCLUSION

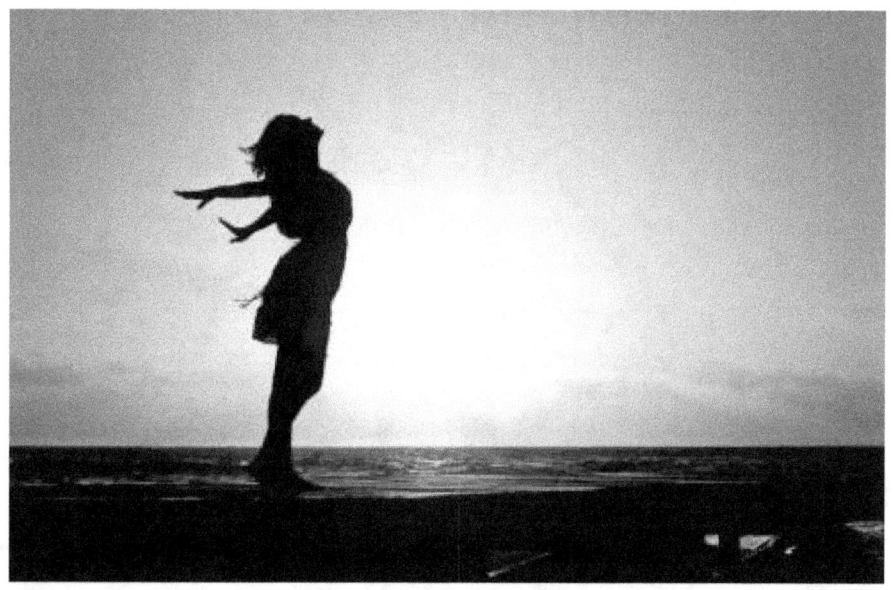

Thank you so much for reading this book, *Intermittent Fasting Over 50: The Ultimate and Complete Guide for Healthy Weight Loss, Burn Fat, Slow Aging, Detox Your Body, and Support Your Hormones with the Process of Metabolic Autophagy*, till the end. Now the best thing for you to do would be to start implementing all the information provided to you in this book. Intermittent fasting will truly change your life for the better. Please don't just read this book and not do anything about it.

We have given you a full proof plan, with recipes and eating schedule. You should have no problem executing it, now go ahead and start bettering your health.

www.ingramcontent.com/pod-product-compliance
Lightning Source LLC
Chambersburg PA
CBHW071806080526
44589CB00012B/713